Eldercare 101

Eldercare 101

A Practical Guide to Later Life Planning, Care, and Wellbeing

Mary Jo Saavedra

in collaboration with
Susan Cain McCarty
Theresa Giddings
Rev. Lawrence Hansen
Dr. Benjamin B. Hellicksn
Joyce Sjoberg and Sara K. Yen

with
Ruth Matinko-Wald, Editor

ROWMAN & LITTLEFIELD
Lanham • Boulder • New York • London

Published by Rowman & Littlefield
A wholly owned subsidiary of The Rowman & Littlefield Publishing Group, Inc.
4501 Forbes Boulevard, Suite 200, Lanham, Maryland 20706
www.rowman.com

Unit A, Whitacre Mews, 26-34 Stannary Street, London SE11 4AB

British Library Cataloguing in Publication Information Available

Library of Congress Cataloging-in-Publication Data

Names: Saavedra, Mary Jo, author.
Title: Eldercare 101 : a practical guide to later life planning, care, and
   wellbeing / Mary Jo Saavedra, Susan Cain McCarty, Theresa Giddings, Rev.
   Lawrence Hansen, Benjamin B. Hellickson, Joyce Sjoberg, Sara K. Yen, and
   Ruth Matinko-Wald.
Description: Lanham : Rowman & Littlefield, [2016]
Identifiers: LCCN 2016006182 (print) | LCCN 2016013469 (ebook) | ISBN
   9781442265462 (cloth : alk. paper) | ISBN 9781442265479 (Electronic)
Subjects: LCSH: Older people—Care. | Caregivers. | Older people—Health and
   hygiene. | Older people—Finance, Personal. | Older people—Religious life.
Classification: LCC HV1451 .S195 2016 (print) | LCC HV1451 (ebook) | DDC
   362.6/3—dc23
LC record available at http://lccn.loc.gov/2016006182

♾™ The paper used in this publication meets the minimum requirements of
American National Standard for Information Sciences—Permanence of Paper
for Printed Library Materials, ANSI/NISO Z39.48-1992.

Printed in the United States of America

This guide is dedicated to my mom,
Dorothy Marie,
and her loving family,
with the blessing that all who use it
will know they are enough.

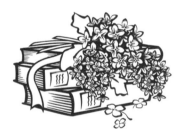

Contents

Preface   ix

Acknowledgments   xiii

Introduction   1

1 LEGAL PILLAR OF AGING WELLBEING   7

Legal Ease   12
Sara K. Yen, JD, LLM

2 FINANCIAL PILLARS OF AGING WELLBEING   29

Money Matters   34
Theresa Giddings, CPA, CFP®
    Getting Organized   35
    Paying the Bills   51
    Insurance   59
    Getting Help with Financial Planning and Advice   66

3 LIVING ENVIRONMENT PILLAR OF WELLBEING   73

Living Environment Options   77
Susan Cain McCarty, MAIS, CSA
    Aging at Home   77
      The Choice   78
      The In-Home Helpers   89
      The Maintenance   98
    Living Options with Built-in Support   103

4   SOCIAL PILLAR OF AGING WELLBEING   117

Social Considerations   122
Susan Cain McCarty, MAIS, CSA
   Life Re-Imagined   122
   Transportation Issues   129
   Managing a Move   134
   Protecting Your Elder   142

5   MEDICAL PILLAR OF AGING WELLBEING   149

Navigating the Medical Maze   154
Joyce Sjoberg, MA, RN, BSN, CMC
   An Ounce of Prevention   155
   Time for Medical Support   164
   Medical Insurance   180
   Geriatric Dentistry / *Benjamin B. Hellickson, DDS*   184
   The Aging Body   191
   Elders and the World of Brain Disease   201
   What to Expect at the End   207

6   SPIRITUAL PILLAR OF AGING WELLBEING   219

Spirituality and the End(s) of Life: Considerations for the
Cared-For and Their Care-Givers   224
Rev. Lawrence Hansen, BCC/CFHPC, CT
   Living Until the End   224
   Dealing with the Dead   234
   Death Dialogue   246
   The Rest Is . . . Spiritual Practices and Poems   251

Glossary   267

Notes   279

Bibliography   283

Index   287

Meet the Authors   293

Preface

This is, without a doubt, a vulnerable time for you as you plan or manage the care of an elder. I know. I have been there. I started managing my mother's care when crisis hit; she had a major fall related to a diagnosis of Alzheimer's disease. I felt numb, hoping someone would hand me a manual, a road map—or simply hold my hand—through this uncharted territory.

Once diagnosed, Mom agreed to move from Seattle to Portland to live near me in a memory care residence. Even with the best facility staff and support of my large family and many friends, I was astonished at all I needed to know and realized I didn't even know all the right questions to ask. Slowly, I painfully pieced together information through endless hours of research. I was riddled with fear, knowing I did not know what I did not know. This made me vulnerable and prone to exhaustion, mistakes, higher costs of care, lost time, and heartache. Oh, did I mention guilt?

Each evening in the early days of her transition to residential care, I held my mother as she cried during states of "sundowners." And I cried with her. I was her youngest of five children. No longer would she pamper and care for me. Gone were the days when this amazing woman would tell me, "Everything is going to be OK."

This period of caring for my mom came as I was finishing my education and thesis in business gerontology. You would think a gerontologist would have all the answers for the care planning and management of an elder, but no, that's not part of our training. However, I didn't need a degree to tell me there were major gaps in eldercare management, and to hope there had to be a better way to navigate the journey.

For six months, I cared for my mother during the day and worked on my graduate thesis at night. Grateful that my amazing family from all corners of the United States were supportive and that my daughter, in her twenties, was strong and independent, I was still constantly mystified as to how to juggle the responsibilities. I had exceptional professionals supporting me and family who helped when I asked. But, still, I faced a seemingly never-ending path of unknowns, crises, and tears. I kept wondering, "How long will this go on?" I was devastated to see my mom suffer and to think this was how we would spend her final days (or would it be years?) together.

In the final week of my mother's life, she was doing well emotionally. We had found a rhythm to our days, and her ability to be present to joy was beginning to expand as her memory slipped further away. She still struggled with scary hallucinations, sundowners, and accelerated decline of memory caused by a change in residence, but we found and cherished grace-filled moments of sharing memories and funny stories. And we were surrounded by a loving, caring community.

Mom was always that "silver lining" kind of woman, filled with faith and with unconditional love for her family. At the beginning of her last week with us, I arrived late one day to the residence home because a dear friend had passed away that morning. My tardiness upset her, and I sensed something had changed. After we went for a walk, she asked if I would stay with her while she took a nap, saying she did not think her pneumonia medicine was working. She fell asleep but within fifteen minutes began to have difficulty breathing. She was under hospice care, so the nurse began comfort measures to help her breathe, hoping the antibiotics would kick in.

Mom declined rapidly that evening. I called my siblings to let them know the end seemed near, and I slept that night on the floor next to her bed. As I listened to her labored breathing, I wondered if I were doing enough. What more would she want of me? She had signed a Physician Orders for Life-Sustaining Treatment (POLST) form stating not to take intervention measures. My tears flowed for all the loss the day had brought. I prayed for God to take my mom swiftly and peacefully so she would not have to suffer any longer if she could not have peace in this world. This had been my prayer most days over the six months, but it usually only made me feel worse, guilty, and that I was not doing enough.

My mother passed a few days later, peacefully, surrounded by her children, my daughter and husband, and a great granddaughter. She was accompanied to her new life on the wings of the prayers of her thirty-four immediate family members, her Carmelite community, and all those who loved her. In her final hours, she left us with a few fleeting moments of consciousness during which she gifted us with a breathtaking smile. At that moment, she was partly in this world and partly in the other. The veil was thin between us and where she was going. In this smile, she shared her joy to be going and her unconditional love for us. All her life she had taught us how to live. Now she also taught us how to die. And she showed us that we were enough and had always been enough.

Two weeks later, I graduated with a master's degree in gerontology. While this was a transformational moment, my grief and my joy commingled with exhaustion. In the following months, the thought burning in my soul, "There has to be a better way," gave rise to a new direction for my postgraduate life. I would become an aging life care manager (ALCM), formerly known as a geriatric care manager (GCM). I had stumbled upon the profession through a teacher during my graduate studies. ALCMs know the magic formulas to assist you when you are in an eldercare crisis. They enable you to catch your breath and continue to walk forward on the path, together with your elder, under their wise guidance.

Why hadn't I heard about ALCMs when my mom was passing? Why did my personal support group and other caregivers in my foxhole of caregiving have no idea these professionals or their services existed and recommend them? Have you heard of ALCMs (or GCMs)? While I learned about them too late to aid me with my mom, I was, nonetheless, sparked to explore how to make a difference in others' caregiving journeys and, two years later, became certified as an ALCM.

Over the years of serving my ALCM clients, I have helped with consultations, crisis management, care planning, care management, and advocacy. And I want you to have the benefit of my knowledge and skills and that of the experts who surround my practice. This is why I created *Eldercare 101*. All the same tools I use for my private clients are in this ready resource. Granted, nothing can replace the skills of hiring an ALCM for private consultation and support, but the basic strategies and solutions in this guide have proven results. They will enable you to successfully help your elder to navigate the Six Pillars of Aging Wellbeing.™ Plus, my hope is that *Eldercare 101* will empower you to thrive, rather than just survive, during your caregiving journey. And I pray that what you learn through *Eldercare 101* will encourage you to fully embrace the blessings you will receive as you give of yourself to another.

Acknowledgments

My deepest thanks go to those who have supported my vision of greater presence for the care and respect of our elders by providing easy access to caregivers for care management information and tools for caregivers. This is sacred work to which we have dedicated ourselves.

To the special people around my table. Jaime, who has taught me to keep walking, one step at a time. You are truly a man of grace and my best friend. My beautiful daughter, Alex Marie, with your tenacious spirit and gentle heart, thank you for walking this path with me. Dorothy and Cy's pride and joy: Kay, Larry and Robin, Neil and Jill, Lance and Yolanda; thank you and your families for teaching me what it is to be family. I am grateful for each of you every day.

To my brilliant collaborators who stepped into my vision with trust and few questions as to where the journey would lead. Susan Cain McCarty, for your partnership in the trenches, creating this better way. Ruthie Matinko-Wald, for your tireless editing and friendly "border collie" nips that made this book come together. To the "wisdom authors" of this book who stepped into the vision of providing a more honoring, empowering, and intentional aging experience for our elders and their caregivers: Susan Cain McCarty, Theresa Giddings, Rev. Larry Hansen, Dr. Ben Hellickson, Joyce Sjoberg, and Sara Yen. Special thanks also go to our generous contributors—especially Donald Altman, Sr. Mary Jo Chaves, Bill Gottlieb, and Kym Croft Miller—for your words of wisdom and encouragement, as well as to our peer editors who answered the call to ensure we had all the dangling threads tightly woven: Susan Cain McCarty, Ruth Cohen, Peggy Kessinger, and Dr. Kathy Masarie.

To those treasures in my life I call friends. Each of you is so dear to me. Thank you also to the following for being an integral part of my own care-giving journey with your life-giving support: Ken, Michael, Sadhana, Poh, Mary, Kym, Marilyn, Sr. Mary Jo, Andrea, Ruth, Pam, Jean, Jim, Francisco, Sr. Cecilia, the Sisters of the Santa Clara Carmelites, and the amazing care-givers at Maryville Memory Care Home. It takes a village.

Introduction

Compassion brings us to a stop,
and for a moment we rise above ourselves.

—Mason Cooley

MARY JO'S FIRESIDE CHAT

So the Journey Begins

Caring for an elder is sacred work. By your commitment as caregiver to an elder person, you participate actively in a good-bye process, acknowledging that life in the physical plane has a natural end. You are that vital companion to another on a one-way journey. And it is you who can ensure that your elder's final years, months, or days are filled with dignity, respect, compassion, meaning, and legacy.

To support you as you care for an elder person, I am thrilled to share with you *Eldercare 101*. You'll find here essential information you need to know. Everything you learn will translate into empowering your elder to live purposefully until the end of his or her natural life and to be valued for his or her important wisdom and gifts. You, ultimately, will be rewarded the gift of saying good-bye in the best way possible.

Our uniquely comprehensive *Eldercare 101* is based on an integrated approach to elder caregiving and is structured upon our Six Pillars of Aging Wellbeing™ process. The six pillars include legal, financial, living environment, social, medical, and spiritual. Full of resources, tips, and management tools, it is a "one-stop shop" for the best and most compassionate advice by experts for common eldercare situations. Used mindfully, *Eldercare 101* can be instrumental in guiding you through the maze of decisions and challenges elders inevitably face.

While many of the twists and turns of eldercare are similar across America, each caregiving situation is unique. You may be planning to help or are already providing care for someone you love deeply. Or you may be caring for someone you are not particularly fond of. You may live in a different city or state from the elder under your care. Is that person a parent, spouse, friend, uncle, or sister? You may be part of a caregiving team together with your siblings, juggling the complex coordination of everyone's opinions. You also may be struggling with less-than-desirable family dynamics or legal issues. Does your particular elder have serious or mild medical complications? Does he or she have cognitive issues? Are you dealing with homecare providers, searching for aging life care team members, or managing the elder's living environment needs?

Chances are, while caring for your elder, you also are trying to maintain your own home, raise children, nurture your relationships with other family members and friends, stay healthy yourself, and perhaps even sustain a professional career. These demands can be undermined by the unpredictable needs of elder caregiving, the time-consuming research it requires, and the crisis that is a constant companion during eldercare.

Whatever your situation, having ready access to the right information will be your greatest asset for effective eldercare planning and crisis management. While caring for my own mom, I carried a binder filled with notes, forms, medical reports, and the like with me at all times. My grab-and-go binder served as a virtual office, file system, and life vault, providing me with the tools I needed at a moment's notice for the coordination of professionals involved in my mom's care. In talking to other caregivers, I learned we all were "reinventing the wheel" of how others had made their caregiving journey easier, better, more informed. We often bounced our way through the maze, hoping to find what we needed for a specific setback or an unexpected crossroad. We commiserated that we felt like deer in headlights with no one place to turn.

Now there is. *Eldercare 101* is that one place for all caregivers and their elders.

The questions you have and the new things you need to learn about eldercare can be overwhelming. Add to that the reality that another's life and resources depend on your getting this right—and guilt, fear, and anxiety can ensue. In fact, guilt could be a nighttime gremlin who dances in your dreams. But there is no room for perfection in caregiving. Humans are involved and the situations are complex, which means caregiving gets messy. Yes, you will make mistakes, but, rest assured: All that is asked of you is that you do your best. You are enough.

As you sort out the complex role of caregiver and embark on your caregiving journey, remember to be gentle with yourself. We suggest you take your first steps with good intention and simply be present to the process. There undoubtedly will be periods of grief for the expected loss of your role as son, daughter, spouse, friend, or partner. To companion with you through your emotions, we have built into *Eldercare 101* guidance and resources to enable you to find calm in the chaos as well as moments of peace and enjoyment.

We know you already possess the heart to meet the life goals of quality, independence, and dignity of your elder. *Eldercare 101* backs up your heart with research-based, expert advice that will shed light along the caregiving tunnel, giving you more clarity and confidence. Buoyed by that confidence, you will take a "do-it-yourself" path and customize your approach to care planning to fit your specific needs and those of your elder.

So, let's get started. As you will soon discover, the first order of business is to surround your elder (and yourself) with support. Our aging life care team diagram on the next page provides a quick snapshot of those you might have on *your* team. Also, the forms listed next are free to download at https://rowman.com/ISBN/9781442265462 and will help you compile your own "grab-and-go" binder for your elder. Take advantage of the many available resources.

Then, serving as your personal aging life care manager, I will lead you through a discussion with six valued professionals. These experts in the Six Pillars of Aging Wellbeing™ will share their experience and provide you with a best-practices framework for the questions, topics, and common situations I see as a care manager. These treasured care management insights ultimately will save you time, money, and heartache. The experts and I also offer you tips, Internet links, and sound care management solutions you can depend on—empowering you to ask the right questions of and speak with knowledge to your own aging life care team of professionals.

Be well,
Mary Jo
Daughter, Mom, Wife, Friend, Gerontologist, Aging Life Care Manager, and Spiritual Director

Aging Life Care Team

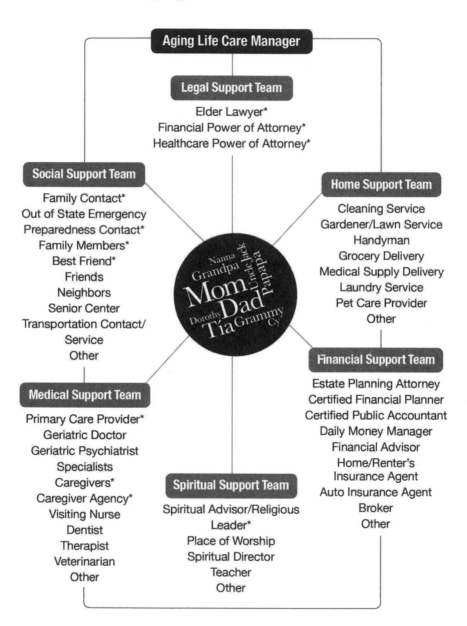

Aging Life Care Manager

Legal Support Team
Elder Lawyer*
Financial Power of Attorney*
Healthcare Power of Attorney*

Social Support Team
Family Contact*
Out of State Emergency
Preparedness Contact*
Family Members*
Best Friend*
Friends
Neighbors
Senior Center
Transportation Contact/
Service
Other

Home Support Team
Cleaning Service
Gardener/Lawn Service
Handyman
Grocery Delivery
Medical Supply Delivery
Laundry Service
Pet Care Provider
Other

Financial Support Team
Estate Planning Attorney
Certified Financial Planner
Certified Public Accountant
Daily Money Manager
Financial Advisor
Home/Renter's
Insurance Agent
Auto Insurance Agent
Broker
Other

Medical Support Team
Primary Care Provider*
Geriatric Doctor
Geriatric Psychiatrist
Specialists
Caregivers*
Caregiver Agency*
Visiting Nurse
Dentist
Therapist
Veterinarian
Other

Spiritual Support Team
Spiritual Advisor/Religious
Leader*
Place of Worship
Spiritual Director
Teacher
Other

For Aging Life Care Team diagrams that can be personalized for your elder and filled in with contact information, go to **http://rowman.com/ISBN/9781442265462.**

*Core Team Members

FREE DOWNLOADABLE FORMS

Available for download at https://rowman.com/ISBN/9781442265462

Aging Life Care Team

Legal Pillar of Aging Wellbeing
Potential Elder Law or Estate Planning Attorneys

Financial Pillar of Aging Wellbeing
Financial Aging Life Care Team
Collectibles Inventory
Strong Box Inventory
Retirement Income: Salaries, Pensions, and Benefits
Individual Retirement Accounts: IRA, Roth IRA, 401(k), and 403(b)
Checking and Savings Accounts
Investments
Credit and Debit Card Accounts
Recurring Payments
Debt Documentation
Cost of Care Worksheet
Documentation of Insurances

Living Environment Pillar of Aging Wellbeing
Potential In-Home Helpers
Potential Adult Foster Care Homes
Potential CCRCs
Potential Assisted Living Facilities
Potential Memory Care Facilities
My Personal Care Team
My Home Team

Social Pillar of Aging Wellbeing
My Village
Potential Adult Day Care Programs
My Possible Rides
My Move Mavens

Medical Pillar of Aging Wellbeing
Medical Aging Life Care Team
Daily Exercise Log

Potential Healthcare Providers
Symptom Tracker
My Medications
Keeping Up with Checkups and Vaccines
Diagnosis List
Record of Medical Visits
Transition Gurus

Spiritual Pillar of Aging Wellbeing
After-Life Considerations for LGBT Elders
After-Life Decision Guide
Planning a Celebration of Life
Writing My Own Obituary

Caregiver Online Communities for Support

AARP Posting Board for Caregivers: http://community.aarp.org/t5/Care
giving/bd-p/bf41?intcmp=AE-HF-IL-COMM-CG
Caregiver Community Sharing Forum: http://eldercare.infopop.cc/6/ubb.x
Caregiver Support Forum: http://www.agingcare.com/Caregiver-Forum
Nurture Yourself: http://www.aarp.org/home-family/caregiving/info-2014/
ways-for-caregivers-to-nurture-themselves.html?intcmp=AE-HF-RELBOX

LEGAL PILLAR OF AGING WELLBEING

In everything, do to others as you would have them do to you;
for this is the essence of the law and the prophets.

—Matthew 7:12

Chapter One

Why Is the Legal Pillar of Aging Wellbeing the First Consideration of Care Management?

My experience as an aging life care manager (ACLM) has proven time and again that the "legal pillar of aging wellbeing" is the best place to start when someone embarks on a caregiving journey with an elder. Legal documents are what empower you to provide the best care and support for your elder. They allow you to understand what your elder wants from you and what she wishes for her end of life.

Caregiving is important and loving work you will want to get right. As you shepherd an elder through the aging experience, you are accompanying her through her final transition. To "get it right" and ensure you help your elder make the best decisions, I highly recommend establishing a relationship with and working through an elder attorney or estate planning attorney, whenever finances permit. Although many do-it-yourself types of legal forms exist, elder lawyers specialize in the complicated issues of advanced aging involving Medicare and Medicaid, estate planning, inheritance, and more.

Initially in the elder aging process, your elder may need only basic legal documents including a will, advance healthcare directive (advance directive), and durable power of attorney (DPOA). Having a professional craft these documents is a good first step toward forging a relationship with a particular attorney. Down the road, when issues arise that require urgent legal counsel, your attorney, as an "aging life care team" member, will be in place to aid your elder—and you, as you begin to take over your elder's legal matters. Over time, the elder lawyer may become a trusted advisor regarding major decisions such as setting up private in-home care, tax considerations, and other legally sensitive topics, or handling issues of concern such as scamming.

In addition to dealing with legal matters that all elders encounter, another area in which elder lawyers can play a major role is mediating family dynamics. For example, a grown child may not like her elder, or vice versa; an elder attorney can recommend formal structures to protect the elder and her assets. Many elders do not have children or family they trust to implement care management and end-of-life wishes. Elder attorneys can work with you to build support systems for your elder for her protection and your peace of mind.

In my aging life care management practice, a common problem occurs when multiple caregivers do not agree on the course of care for a parent. One of my cases, for example, involved a family of five children and two living parents in their eighties. The father of the children, Ed, had Alzheimer's disease. The mother, Katherine, could no longer care for Ed herself, because of her own failing health.

After initial conversations with the entire family, I began the assessment process. Both Ed and Katherine identified their needs and wants, they assessed their resources and support options, and each of the children outlined his and her own goals to help Ed and Katherine understand that safety and security had to dovetail with their parents' desire for a quality life. I then helped the family create a care plan that would best provide for the parents—with the priority of keeping Ed and Katherine together for as long as possible.

When I interviewed Katherine, I concluded that she was exhausted and tired of arguing with some of the children over the next steps. She also was stressed emotionally from watching her husband of fifty-two years slip away before her eyes. She had wanted to live out her life with Ed under the care of others at a place where she could live alongside him, share meals, and continue to experience special times together. To help her accomplish her goals, she had appointed one of her sons to be their power of attorney (POA), to oversee their care plan, and to serve as the main contact for her and her husband's aging life care team. Although she said she would consider all the siblings' input when decisions needed to be made, this son would, ultimately, carry out the decisions.

During the first few months the son was acting in the role of care manager, everything was going well. Ed had settled into a memory care facility after a few weeks of rough transition, and Katherine was regaining some of her health and strength. The family had put together an impressive aging life care team to support them, both Ed and Katherine were getting the medical care they needed, and their social and spiritual needs were being met. Soon thereafter, however, I received a call from the son. He shared that his siblings were calling into question his POA authority regarding their father, and, in short time, each child had a lawyer representing his and her positions.

The situation gravely distressed Katherine. I could see she was sinking under the stress of her sadness. One of the children was even threatening to have Katherine declared incompetent. At this point, I consulted with Katherine, her doctor, and her elder attorney. The elder attorney recommended a mediation process to explore a third-party guardianship for Ed. Through the process, all siblings and Katherine expressed their concerns and acknowledged their deep grief regarding the father's situation. One of the sons admitted he was simply unable to see his dad in decline and living in a locked facility. The mediation process allowed for the validation of each child's voice and for Katherine to express her love in a way each needed to hear. Appeased, everyone agreed to the third-party guardianship, and the children restored their individual relationships with their parents. This also minimized the challenges of the group-decision dynamics.

This real-life family scenario highlights a common struggle for adults acting as caregivers for their parents. When health and ability decline, elders can become dependent on their children, reversing the traditional parent-child role. Most grown children navigate this new role out of sheer determination, but, too often and without realizing it, they grieve the loss of the parent while the elder is still alive. If you are in this situation, know this sense of loss is natural, is expected, and marks the beginning of the process of letting go of your parent. Having the help of an elder attorney—as well as an aging life care manager—can take off some of the pressure, allowing you to find windows of time to feel like your parent's child again. These windows provide moments for being present to the end-of-life needs of a parent or loved one, and a space to savor the time you have together.

In chapter 1, elder lawyer and estate planning attorney Sara Yen defines legal terms and outlines the necessary legal documents and legal needs of elders. She also highlights some special considerations within the legal system for elders. All this information provides a strong framework to use as the basis for a discussion with your own elder or an elder lawyer.

Legal Ease

Sara K. Yen, JD, LLM

As we age, we have lots of legal planning to do—from setting up a POA to drawing up a will or trust to planning how to divide up what we will leave behind. Professional legal services can help everyone make the most of a legacy built over a lifetime and can provide guiding advice to your loved ones regarding their care and end-of-life wishes. Although the idea of working with an attorney to address some of the legal issues we face can sometimes be intimidating or overwhelming, working with the *right* attorney, one who focuses on serving elders, is usually a wise decision.

In an effort to help ease the effort of learning about and doing all the legal necessities, the information compiled here will prove invaluable. Please note, however, that the information in this text is intended to provide general guidance rather than advice specific for any particular situation. Because the law is dynamic, and because the outcome of any given case requires the application of unique facts to the law, the information in this book is not intended to serve as legal, accounting, investment, or tax advice. You, therefore, should not act upon any information in this book or chapter without first consulting legal counsel directly. Also note that use of this book or chapter does not create an attorney-client relationship.

ATTORNEYS FOR ELDERS

Two main types of attorneys provide services for elders and their families: elder law attorneys and estate planning attorneys. Because "elder law" and "estate planning" overlap to a great degree, many lawyers who work with elders include both types of services in their practices.

Elder Law Attorneys

- Focus on cases and legal work involving elders.
- Services vary and include guardianship and conservatorship cases, elder abuse cases, and the like.
- Some elder law attorneys focus on Medicaid and other needs-based public benefits planning. Most Medicaid planning attorneys also handle guardianships and conservatorships. Those who focus on Medicaid may not directly handle litigation, but they often can be a good referral source for a litigation attorney, if an elder abuse or an elder litigation issue arises.

Estate Planning Attorneys

- Create plans to address proper management of assets and healthcare decisions in the event of incapacity (i.e., the lack of ability to care for oneself).
- Facilitate the distribution of assets at the end of life (e.g., transferring property to the next generations, charitable planning, expressing preferences regarding extraordinary life support measures and healthcare decisions, and addressing potential estate tax issues).
- Help guide families through probate, estate, and trust administration, which can be a time-consuming, emotional, and confusing process.

Alternatives to Using an Attorney?

Self-drafting programs, such as the online Legal Zoom at www.legalzoom.com, are an alternative to using (and paying for) an attorney. Keep in mind, however, that these programs are, by necessity, created to be "all things to all people" and often will not address the specifics of an individual's situation. Additionally, though they claim you do not need a lawyer, they recommend you have their documents reviewed by an attorney.

Finding the Right Attorney

To find an elder law or estate planning attorney in your area, start by asking for referrals from your family, friends, and the other professionals with whom you work. If you have a financial advisor, accountant, or aging life care manager, she will frequently refer you to a qualified attorney. Also, you can search online for "elder law or estate planning attorney [your state]" and you will find websites listing lawyers in your area; these websites provide contact information on each attorney and occasionally include reviews from former clients. In addition, many state bar associations will have a lawyer referral service. You can find your state bar association by searching online for "[your state] bar association." Once you have a referral or an attorney in mind, be sure to review her website to have a sense of her fees and how she approaches working with clients. Here are a few websites with which to begin your search:

http://www.avvo.com
http://www.estateplanning.com
http://www.findlaw.com
http://www.naela.org

National Resources

American Bar Association: http://www.americanbar.org/groups/real_property_
  trust_estate/resources/estate_planning.html
ElderCounsel: http://www.eldercounsel.com/
National Academy of Elder Law Attorneys: http://www.naela.org/
National Elder Law Foundation: http://www.nelf.org/
WealthCounsel: http://www.estateplanning.com/ and http://www.elderlaw
  answers.com/

Online Communities

Lawyers.com: http://community.lawyers.com/forums/default.aspx?GroupID=
17. This online forum focuses on wills, trusts, and estates.
Avvo.com: http://www.avvo.com. Through this website, attorneys will answer questions posted online. Please keep in mind that the responses on this
forum may not be from an attorney in your state; a local attorney should be
consulted for confirmation of any online response.

For a form to keep track of referrals for **"Potential Elder Law or Estate Planning Attorneys,"** go to https://rowman.com/ISBN/9781442265462.

LEGALESE DEFINED

Once you have an elder law or estate planning attorney, these are the documents and terms you'll be discussing. If, even after reviewing these definitions, you don't understand something, never be afraid to ask your attorney.

Advance Healthcare Directive (or Advance Directive): Gives instructions
for future life-sustaining treatment and typically includes a HCPOA, which
names the "healthcare agent" who will make healthcare decisions for an
individual in the event the individual is unable to communicate.
   Each state typically will have its own statutory document that should be
used. If your state uses a statutory document (meaning a document that is
always in a particular form under state law), you often can get this from
your doctor. Also, most estate planning and elder law attorneys include this
form for their clients as part of their overall planning process.
   All adults, regardless of their current health status, are recommended to
complete this document. **Keep it with the rest of your estate planning
documents (your trust, will, and DPOA). Giving a copy to your pri-**

mary care provider is a good idea. This document will *not* guide emergency medical personnel, but the document does guide inpatient treatment decisions if it is available.

An advance healthcare directive is sometimes confused with a living will. They are similar documents in that both give instructions regarding life-sustaining treatment, but the advance healthcare directive also typically includes the HCPOA in the document. If your state uses a living will, you probably also will need to complete a separate HCPOA. You should consult with your estate planning attorney regarding what documents are required and appropriate in your state. You can download your state's advance directive by visiting http://www.caringinfo.org.

Beneficiary: A person named to receive property after the death of the property owner. A beneficiary is typically named in a last will and testament, a trust, in a beneficiary designation on a retirement account or insurance policy, or in a "Transfer on Death" or "Payable on Death" designation on certain types of financial accounts. *Note*: A beneficiary designation overrides a will.

Conservator: A person appointed by a court to take care of the finances of a "protected person," who is someone the court has determined needs assistance with the management of finances and assets. Most conservators are family members, or sometimes friends, who agree to serve. There are also professionals who will serve in this capacity, or they can be appointed by the court, if there is no family member or friend willing or able to serve.

Conservatorship: A matter in which a court-appointed individual, the "conservator," takes care of the financial and legal matters of someone the court deems needs assistance with such management. A conservatorship is typically required when someone becomes incapacitated and does not have proper planning in place (a DPOA or a trust), which would allow her assets to be managed on her behalf without court intervention. The court is required to be involved at that point in order for someone to have legal authority to manage the incapacitated person's assets.

Decedent: A person who has died.

Durable Power of Attorney (DPOA): A document in which someone, "the principal," names an "agent" or "attorney-in-fact" to manage her assets and finances. This can be created to be effective immediately or to have effect upon incapacity (a "springing" POA). A DPOA no longer has any legal effect after the death of the principal. A DPOA can be drafted by your estate planning or elder law attorney to address your specific situation.

Estate: All property and debts belonging to a person. Everyone has an "estate," regardless of size.

Executor, Personal Representative, or Administrator: A person named in a last will and testament (personal representative or executor) or appointed by a court (administrator) to oversee the administration of the estate of someone who has passed away. An administrator is appointed by the court when the decedent did not have a last will and testament. There are many considerations that go into choosing the appropriate person to serve as personal representative. Your estate planning attorney should guide you through this choice when you are designing your estate plan.

Fiduciary: A person who has a legal duty to act solely in another party's interest. A personal representative, executor, administrator, trustee, conservator, guardian, healthcare agent, and attorney-in-fact are all types of fiduciaries.

Guardianship: A matter in which a court-appointed and supervised individual, the "guardian," makes day-to-day decisions for a "protected person," someone the court has determined needs assistance with those decisions due to the potential for harm to herself or others, most often due to incapacity or some other cognitive impairment. The appointed guardian is responsible for decisions such as living situations, management of health care, or advance funeral arrangements. A guardianship is typically required when someone becomes incapacitated and does not have proper planning in place (HCPOA, HIPAA authorization, advance healthcare directive), which would allow another person to manage the care of the incapacitated person without court intervention.

Healthcare Power of Attorney (HCPOA): A document in which an "agent" is named to make healthcare decisions for an individual, the "principal." If you are in a state that uses an advance healthcare directive, the HCPOA is typically included in that document. Otherwise, your estate planning attorney should include this document in your estate plan.

Healthcare Representative or Healthcare Agent: This is a person named in an advance directive or a HCPOA to manage the healthcare decisions of the principal in the event she is unable to communicate or is otherwise incapacitated.

Health Insurance Portability and Accountability Act (HIPAA): This act was passed by Congress in 1996; it limits access to private healthcare information. A properly drafted estate plan should include a HIPAA authorization and release, so the principal's loved ones can have access to necessary medical information.

Heir: A person legally entitled to inherit assets of a decedent, based on state statute and when there is no other planning in place, such as a will or trust. For example, a child is typically an heir of her widowed father. If the father has no estate plan (i.e., no will or trust), the child will inherit based on the laws of intestacy in the state where the father lived. The father can, however, disinherit the child or include additional beneficiaries if he creates a last will and testament or a trust in which he specifies how he wants his assets to be distributed.

Incapacity: A lack or the loss of the ability to take care of oneself.

Intestacy: Intestacy means, simply, dying without having a will in place. The practical result of intestacy is that state statute will determine where and to whom the assets will pass. This may or may not match the wishes of the decedent. For example, James Dean's estate passed to the long-estranged father who abandoned him, because he had no will or trust in place.

Last Will and Testament: A legal document that names beneficiaries of property of a decedent and a person responsible for overseeing the distribution of the property. The responsible person is called an "executor" or "personal representative." Wills only have legal effect at death.

Living Will: *See* Advance Healthcare Directive.

Ombudsman: Professional who advocates for residents of long-term care facilities. Each state's ombudsman can typically be found by searching online for "ombudsman [state]." States also require that the ombudsman's name and contact information be posted in plain sight in adult care facilities.

Personal Representative (PR): *See* Executor.

Physician Orders for Life-Sustaining Treatment (POLST): This is a companion to an advance healthcare directive or a living will, intended for persons of any age who have a serious illness. The POLST gives medical orders for current treatment and will guide inpatient treatment. Unlike the advance directive or a living will, the POLST *will* guide emergency medical personnel, if it is available.

Currently, POLST forms are available in more than half of the states in the United States, and they use various names—MOLST, POST, and COLST. To learn about the POLST form in your state or to find out if your state is developing one, check out http://www.polst.org/programs-in-your-state. In states where they are available, POLST forms can be obtained from primary care physicians, who must sign and register the form in the POLST national database. POLST forms are typically required to be printed on a specific color of paper. Also, post the complete POLST form in a public location such as the refrigerator, so it is easily accessible in the event of an emergency.

Power of Attorney (POA): A legal document giving someone the authority to sign documents and conduct transactions on another person's behalf. POAs are common estate planning documents; many people sign a financial power of attorney, also known as a durable power of attorney (DPOA), to give a friend or family member the power to conduct financial transactions for them if they become incapacitated. People also commonly sign healthcare powers of attorney (HCPOA) to give someone else the authority to make medical decisions if they are unable to do so. You also might give someone POA to act in a particular transaction if you cannot do it yourself, such as signing documents at a real estate closing when you are out of town.

Probate: The process of settling a decedent's estate under the supervision of a court. Probate is necessary if someone dies without an estate plan in place, or if she passes away with a will-only plan (i.e., no trust in place).

Trust: A private legal document that controls the management of property and assets during each stage of life—while alive and well, during incapacity, and at death. A trust is a contract, and it takes effect immediately upon signing. Assets in a properly drafted, funded, and maintained trust will avoid having to go through the probate process, which often can save families time, money, and hassle.

Trustee: A trustee is the person in charge of protecting, managing, and distributing the assets held in a trust. A successor trustee is the person who will step in to serve if the initial trustee cannot or will not serve.

FIRST THINGS FIRST: COMPILE IMPORTANT DOCUMENTS

One of the first places to start in helping elders to put their legal affairs in order is to assist them in compiling their important documents. Among the first they should have accessible are:

- **Durable (or Financial) Power of Attorney** (also referred to as DPOA)
- **Healthcare (or Medical) Power of Attorney** (also referred to as HCPOA)
- **Physician Orders for Life-Sustaining Treatment** (POLST)
- **Advance Healthcare Directive** (or Advance Directive)

If you are the primary caregiver of an elder who has not officially designated you as her agent in a DPOA or healthcare agent in a HCPOA, have your elder visit with an attorney to sign the forms. Without these documents, you will not be able to advocate on behalf of your loved one, let alone even have a doctor or other professional speak to you regarding your elder, without going to court to obtain a guardianship or conservatorship. Be aware that the attorney who is writing these documents for your elder represents the elder, not you, and will take direction from your elder regarding the content of the documents.

Other documents that should be located and compiled for reference and safekeeping are:

- Will/Trust
- Birth certificate
- Military discharge records
- Social security card
- Passport

- House deed
- Other real estate deeds and titles
- Title transfers
- Car title and registration
- RV, boat, and other recreational vehicle titles and registration
- HIPAA Authorization and Release
- For Executor: Death certificate/record

Now Secure Them!

Once the documents are located, be sure to secure them in a designated place. Keeping all important documents in, for example, a home safe or in a safety deposit box at the bank is a good protection from fire and theft. However, safe deposit boxes can be difficult to access, depending on the financial institution. Consider having the POA agent or a family member have signature authority on any safe deposit box. Be sure to confirm the POA's ability to access the box while the elder is alive and well. Keep the copies and keys in a portable file and ensure family members or agents under DPOA know where the copies and keys are. (See the "Financial" section on safe deposit boxes for more information and tips.)

Special Note: Keep the POLST and advance directive highly accessible.

Do not keep the advance healthcare directive and POLST in the home safe or security box, as the originals of these documents must be easily accessible to caregivers and emergency medical technicians. Some people place these documents in a ziplock bag or other protective covering and tape them to the refrigerator door or some other very visible location.

INVENTORY YOUR ASSETS

Before an estate plan can be established, an inventory of assets must be completed. An estate planning attorney must have a good picture of how much an estate is worth, what debts exist, what kinds of assets make up the estate, and how those assets are owned before she can provide good legal advice regarding the design of an estate plan. Likewise, an elder law attorney needs a complete inventory of assets to determine potential eligibility for Medicaid benefits.

In the case of someone becoming incapacitated, the fiduciary stepping in to assist (agent under a DPOA, successor trustee, or conservator) needs an inventory of assets to determine what steps to take in the management of those assets. Also, at death, an inventory of assets is needed to determine proper estate and trust administration procedures.

What estate planning attorneys are looking for:

- Current list of assets
- How they are titled
- Appropriate person or firm to contact regarding the asset
- Current beneficiaries named on the account, including any "Transfer on Death" or "Payable on Death" designation
- What large gifts have been made previously and whether a gift tax return was filed
- Any existing estate planning documents (DPOA, trust, will, healthcare documents)

In the "Financial" section of this publication, your elder will be guided to create an inventory of her assets. We also recommend she designate an agent in a DPOA, share the information gathered with that individual, and give her the authority to watch over all legal and financial affairs when she cannot or when she no longer wants the burden. We cannot stress enough that asking for help is a very smart move, especially when dealing with legal and money matters!

Be Sure to Review Beneficiary Designations

A review of beneficiary designations can prevent unintended consequences from outdated designations. This will help ensure your elder's plan is still valid and will accomplish her desired outcome. A good estate planning or elder law attorney will always determine the current beneficiary designations on accounts and recommend any necessary changes as part of the planning process. *The designated beneficiary on any account or policy overrides any gift or distribution in a will or trust*; therefore, make sure that records regarding these accounts and policies are up to date. Beneficiary designations cannot be changed once someone becomes incapacitated, absent a valid DPOA which authorizes the agent to make beneficiary changes and change estate planning. Your elder should ask her estate planning attorney whether her DPOA contains these necessary provisions, if she would like her agent to be authorized to make changes to the estate plan if she becomes incapacitated.

Other Asset Tips

- **Keep good records** of all financial transactions, and let "helpers" know where these records can be found.
- **Make sure any trusts are "funded."** That is, make sure accounts are properly titled in the name of the trust and have the correct beneficiary designa-

tions to fit the design of the plan. An unfunded trust will not do what it is intended to do, and the plan is broken until the trust is funded.

- **Keep a list of passwords and log-in information for all digital assets** including e-mail accounts, social network accounts, online banking accounts, etc. Having a list or one place to look is handy to avoid the headache of having access to those accounts denied to agents/personal representatives after death.

Go to https://rowman.com/ISBN/9781442265462 for **"Getting Organized"** forms.

There's an App for That!

For password management and online file storage, check out these online apps that allow you to develop, safely store, and easily access hundreds of passwords and other information such as driver's license and passport data or credit card and loan numbers. With these apps, you only have to remember one single master password or select a key file to unlock your whole database. Note that you should have many passwords for all your online social networking, banking, e-commerce, or investment activities. If you use the same password over and over, you are in danger of being hacked!

1Password: www.1password.com
KeePass: http://keepass.info/
Keeper: https://keepersecurity.com/
LastPass: https://lastpass.com/

THE FOUNDATIONAL ESTATE DOCUMENT: WILLS AND REVOCABLE TRUSTS

If your elders already have a will or a revocable trust, great! If they do not, you will want to suggest they have an estate planning or elder law attorney draft a will or trust for them as their foundational or main estate planning document. They might also consider using an online drafting program such as Legal Zoom, but be aware they may get one-size-fits-all documents with such programs, and they will not have the benefits of the advice and experience of a good attorney. In either case, they will want to know the pros and cons of wills and trusts.

Wills

- **CON:** Assets will require a probate to be distributed if you only have a will.
  - Probate is costly.
  - Probate is time-consuming.
  - Probate is a public proceeding.
  - Probate process is controlled by the judge and court.
- **CON:** Will has no legal effect until death; that is, it cannot include lifetime (i.e., incapacity) planning.
- **CON:** If you have assets in more than one state, you will need a probate in each state where the property is located.
- **PRO:** Usually will cost less than a revocable trust to draft with an attorney.

Revocable Trusts

- **CON:** Typically will cost more to draft with an attorney.
- **CON:** Moving assets into the trust can sometimes be time-consuming (but it only has to be done once for each asset).
- **PRO:** Takes effect upon signing, so is an excellent vehicle to handle incapacity. A successor trustee can step in very easily and smoothly in a properly drafted trust, which allows continued management of finances and assets without court intervention.
- **PRO:** Administration upon death does not require probate, which means it is private, typically less costly, faster, and controlled by the terms of the trust, not the court.
- **PRO:** If there is property in more than one state that has been moved into the trust, a single administration can handle the distribution of all trust property.

Things to Think about Ahead of Time

Who Will Inherit the Assets?

Your elders will need to determine who will inherit their estate (assets) when they pass away. Will it all go to a spouse? Will it go to children? In equal shares, or with different percentages? Will they include their sons- or daughters-in-law? Should they make provisions to protect the inheritance of a child from potential divorce?

How Will the Heirs Inherit?

Will they receive the assets outright (i.e., "cash in hand")? Should some or all receive the assets instead in an ongoing trust?

What Happens If a Beneficiary Dies Before Your Elders Do?

Once beneficiaries have been chosen, your elders should decide what happens if any of the beneficiaries predecease them. If assets are going to a child who predeceases them, will that child's share go to his or her children (the grandchildren)? Also, your elders will want to determine their remote contingent beneficiary(ies)—that person or persons who would receive the assets if all other named beneficiaries die before your elders. For example, should the assets go to siblings, nieces and nephews, dear friends? Perhaps a charity or other organization?

Are There Any Family Heirlooms or Personal Items Your Elders Wish to Go to Specific Persons? Other Gifts?

Do they have any gifts they would like to make? This is where they would make a gift to an organization they support, or to a friend or other family member they wish to honor.

FOUR SPECIAL LEGAL ISSUES

Are You in a Same-Sex Relationship?

Unmarried same-sex couples should be sure to complete estate planning documents granting their partner decision-making authority, when desired, for healthcare and finances. The federal and state laws surrounding partnership, registered domestic partnership, and marriage for same-sex couples are very fluid. Be sure to check with your planning attorney regarding these issues, as well as the current status of the law in your state and on a federal level. Regardless of what changes occur in the laws, couples will want to put in place planning strategies to protect themselves, their partner or spouse, their children, and other loved ones. For same-sex couples, naming an agent in both a DPOA and a HCPOA is especially important. Laws differ in each state, so, if partners wish to make crucial financial and healthcare decisions for each other, these documents must be completed with an experienced estate planning attorney.

Potentially Eligible for Medicaid or Another Need-Based Public Benefit Program?

If there is any possibility your elder may apply to receive Medicaid benefits, *do not* contact any Medicaid office, even for basic information, before having a consultation with a Medicaid planning attorney, as any contact with the agency may affect what rights and authority the agency has regarding your situation.

To qualify for need-based public benefit programs including Medicaid, applicants must meet certain financial and health requirements, but the rules can be complicated and are constantly changing. In fact, many "myths" are afloat, and falling into a trap without being fully advised of the options can be a costly mistake. With the help of a Medicaid planning attorney who knows your state's specific rules and who can recommend how to structure your elder's assets and income, your elder might qualify for benefits for which she might not otherwise have qualified. Money spent on a will or trust before exploring Medicaid as an option could be an expensive mistake.

Have a Medically Embedded Device?

If your elder has a medically embedded device, such as a pacemaker or an implantable cardioverter-defibrillator (ICD), consider whether she should give instructions in an advance directive or POLST regarding if or when the device should be turned off or deactivated. The agent named in the document will ultimately direct this decision, but providing direction to the agent can help remove a heavy burden from the agent surrounding that decision. Having prior written direction also potentially can head off any ethical struggles with a medical facility. Please keep in mind that a medical facility's ethics decisions may be influenced by other factors, such as a whether the facility has a faith-based mission along with its healthcare mission. (See our "Spiritual" section for more on this issue.)

What about Pets?

Many people worry about what will happen to their pets. In some states, arrangements can be made for the care of beloved pets with pet trusts, which are designed to name caregivers and designate funds for the benefit of pets in case of the loss of their owner. Leaving detailed information about how to best care for the pet, the pet owner can have peace of mind that her furry friends won't suffer after her death. For more information, visit https://www.aspca.org/pet-care/planning-for-your-pets-future/pet-trust-primer. (Also, see our "Living Environment" section for more on this issue.)

FAQS TO REVIEW WITH YOUR ELDER

What Happens If I Don't Have a Will or Trust?

Your property will be distributed according to your state's intestacy laws. These may include individuals you do *not* want to inherit (e.g., an estranged family member) and may not include someone you *do* want to benefit (e.g., a close friend, unmarried partner, stepchild).

Should I Worry about Probate?

As noted earlier, probate is the process of settling a decedent's estate under the supervision of a court when that person dies without an estate plan in place, or if she passes away with a will-only plan (i.e., no trust in place). The probate process varies from state to state, and the process in some states is better or worse than in others. The concerns most individuals have about probate are:

- Probate is a public proceeding; anyone can get information on an open probate file.
- Probate is controlled by the court.
- Probate can be time-consuming and lengthy.
- Probate can be expensive.
- Probate can be frustrating for the surviving family members.

How Do We Best Prepare for a Medical Emergency?

Keep the original advance healthcare directive or living will and a copy of the POLST in a place that is easily accessible in the event of a medical emergency. And keep the original POLST and a copy of the advance healthcare directive or living will posted on the refrigerator. Speak to your caregivers and loved ones about your wishes in the event of an emergency. Be sure they know who your medical providers are and how to contact them.

How Do We Best Protect Originals while Keeping Them Accessible?

You might store your original legal and financial documents in a fireproof safe, sharing the combination with the appropriate people or having a key stored in a designated location. An alternative is a safe deposit box that can be opened by a future trustee or personal representative, although gaining access to boxes in an emergency situation can sometimes be difficult. (See more about this in our "Financial" section.)

Who Is Best Suited for the Role of POA?

Choosing the right people for each role is essential and differs for each individual. Keep in mind that the person chosen is granted authority over your assets or your person, and she must be someone you trust without hesitation. A skillful and experienced estate planning attorney can help guide you to the right choice. An aging life care manager might also be able to help you choose.

Who Can Help Handle Settling the Various Accounts and Debts?

An estate planning, probate, or trust administration attorney will help guide your personal representative or trustee through the administration process including dealing with creditors, any required court process such as probate, working with an accountant regarding final income and estate tax returns, and, ultimately, distributing estate assets.

What about the Final Tax Returns?

A qualified accountant will work with your probate/trust administration attorney to timely file any required state and federal income and estate tax returns.

CHECKLIST FOR POST-DEATH OF A LOVED ONE

Things to Do Right Away

- Determine if there is any property that needs to be protected, such as a vacant rental house or vehicle. Protect property against loss from theft or vandalism.
- Ensure that proper funeral arrangements are made, and that *the funeral home orders at least ten death certificates from the state.* You may need an official death certificate to proceed with each legal or financial matter.

Things to Do within Two Weeks

- Locate original will or trust. Do not write on the original documents.
- Locate important records, such as account statements, titles and deeds, and life insurance policies.
- Choose an attorney to work with on the estate administration and make an appointment. Bring all original estate planning documents (will, trust, etc.) to the meeting, along with all financial information gathered to date.
- Notify insurance and annuity companies of the death and request claim forms.
- If mortgage life insurance on home exists, notify insurance company.
- Determine what creditors exist and whether any must be paid immediately.
- Cancel credit cards in your elder's name.
- Change delivery of mail to proposed trustee or personal representative or to administration attorney's office.

Things to Do within One Month

- Notify the Social Security Administration and any other organization that pays annuity or retirement funds. Be aware that direct deposits already made from these organizations will likely be returned.
- Gather and organize financial documents.
  - Bank statements
  - Brokerage and other investment account statements
  - Stock certificates
  - Bond certificates
  - Promissory notes
  - Titles to vehicles
  - Deeds to real property
  - Appraisals on any valuable personal property
- Access and inventory safe deposit box.

For printable, easy-to-fill-in forms for keeping track of all documents, go to https://rowman.com/ISBN/9781442265462.

FINANCIAL PILLAR OF AGING WELLBEING

The greatest treasures are those invisible to the eye and found by the heart.

—Buddha

Chapter Two

MARY JO'S FIRESIDE CHAT

Money: The Most Common Pillar with Which Aging Adults Need Help

Money complicates everything. Having it creates options for an elder's wellbeing, but not having it can destabilize his wellbeing—and that of his loved ones. The questions surrounding money matters related to the elderly are endless: Will his money last until he dies? How are his assets best protected? Are the siblings fighting over who gets what? Who is going to pay the bills? What is a good estate strategy? Will the long-term care insurance pay for living in an adult foster home? How can I help Mom and Dad if they won't talk to me? I don't have children, so to whom do I turn for financial help? And the questions go on!

On top of financial issues just being plain complex, money is often an emotional hotbed. For example, the cost of sustained care in the elder years and having to make a financial decision to move the elder to a new residence can be quite painful. In some cultures, discussing a parent's financial situation openly is considered inappropriate. In other families, a parent may not feel safe disclosing his financial status to a particular grown child who is offering to help. And, if the elder has limited resources, perhaps a grown child is paying for eldercare but still needs to protect his own assets. In these sticky situations, having professional help is smart. In fact, financial management can be tamed by introducing the right aging life care team members and putting security measures in place that honor the elder's wishes. For example, an ALCM can help find benefits that may have been overlooked to supplement an elder's own resources, and a credentialed financial advisor can help manage an elder's assets. If your elder already has his DPOA in place and all is well, checking in with your financial aging life care team members annually will ensure the finances stay well.

If your role is financial POA for your elder, having a clear snapshot of your elder's current financial situation is critical. You need to know what systems need to be managed and understand what safeguards need to be put in place to protect against scamming and even abuse. When I first started my aging life care management practice, a successful entrepreneur, Rebecca, called for my help. She and her husband, Troy, were concerned that her father's new wife might be stealing money from his estate.

Rebecca's dad, Ben, was eighty-five at the time. Troy had managed Ben's finances until he remarried five years earlier, when Ben's new wife took over the finances. The first few years of Ben's new marriage seemed wonderful, and Rebecca and Troy were thrilled to see Ben so happy. Then Ben's health began to decline rapidly due to memory loss. When Rebecca and Troy visited with Ben, they would notice his appearance was disheveled, he was not eating well, and a few valuables were gone from the home. In addition, Ben's wife began to ask Rebecca to help pay for Ben's care, although Rebecca knew Ben had an extensive estate and did not need her financial help. Quickly, Rebecca's relationship with the wife became estranged and worrisome.

Over a period of six months, Rebecca and Troy became very concerned for Ben's wellbeing and observed that his wife was behaving more and more erratically. They decided to bring in the police to investigate and called me to learn what else they might do to protect Ben. We talked over Ben's health decline and his wife's health, identified the main concerns that fueled their worries, assessed if Rebecca had POA for Ben (which luckily she did), and set in motion immediate action to ensure Ben's wellbeing. I also recommended that Rebecca bring in a forensic accountant. The accountant reconstructed Ben's finances for the past five years, and he found clear evidence of financial abuse starting at the beginning of Ben and his wife's relationship. Rebecca and Troy's worst fears were confirmed, and they proceeded to press criminal charges against Ben's wife.

Financial exploitation of elders comes in many forms—from internal family threats as well as from external threats from strangers (e.g., door-to-door, e-mail, and phone-call scams). In addition, elders are at high risk of their own mismanagement of money because of illness, adverse reaction to medication, and changes in cognitive abilities. Because of the increase in financial risk as people age, we highly recommend establishing formal financial systems— such as automated bill paying—starting at age sixty or sooner. Having sound financial systems in place early on can sustain security and ensure more successful transitions into older age.

The place to begin in setting up financial systems that will withstand the pressures elders face is by hiring a financial advisor such as a wealth manager, a Certified Financial Planner™ (CFP®), a certified public accountant (CPA), a daily money manager (DMM), or other trusted aging life care team members. By building relationships in younger years with any of these financial professionals, elders will have expert help to guide them through the more complex needs that arise in later years. In addition, having an aging life care team member who is a trusted DPOA can aid in the management of these professionals, help to reduce your elder's financial risk, and ensure best use of resources needed for the elder's care. This type of team approach allows you to have several sets of eyes guiding and guarding the financial wellbeing of your elder—with confidentiality—whether you live next door or in a different state.

For the "Financial" section of *Eldercare 101*, I have asked CPA and CFP® Theresa Giddings to explain the tools of money matters related to elders. She addresses specific financial management strategies, resource options, pitfalls, insurance, financial terms, and financial documents. She also highlights what one should consider before selling a family home to pay for care as well as how to protect elders from scamming threats. All this information will provide you with a strong framework to use as the basis for a discussion with your elder—and his financial aging life care team members.

Money Matters

Theresa Giddings, CPA, CFP®

One of the biggest headaches for most people as they age is dealing with money matters. Do I have enough to live comfortably for the rest of my life? What happens if I become ill or incapacitated? What do I need to know about my finances in the event I outlive my partner who's been taking care of our finances for our entire married lives? Do I need an accountant? Should I refinance my mortgage? Do I need to establish a financial POA? If I have long-term care insurance, what does it really cover? What happens to my estate when I pass away? The questions can be endless and overwhelming. You might not even know all the questions you should ask!

In this section of *Eldercare 101*, we spell out the ABCs of financial management. The main topics include:

- Getting Organized
- Paying the Bills
- Insurance
- Getting Help with Financial Planning and Advice

Each of the four sections features tips, products, and programs that will help you to help your elder make sound financial decisions and stay on top of financial responsibilities. We conclude the section with a "Financial Glossary" and a "Ready Reference for Financial Contacts," where you can find websites and phone numbers for various financial services. By the time you finish working through this section of *Eldercare 101*, we hope you and the elders for whom you are caring will be on your way to feeling more confident about money matters through the "golden years."

If working through this section makes your elders uneasy, you might consider recommending that they ask one of their children (you?) or a trusted friend (you?) to be their DPOA. To do so, the elders can show that person this section of *Eldercare 101* and ask if he would be willing to assist in gathering information, assessing needs, or maybe even taking over bill paying. If the person accepts the invitation, then, as noted in our "Legal" section, your elders would contact an attorney and fill out a form that legally gives that person the authority as the DPOA. An ALCM also can help to initiate the conversation or help to find the right professional to advise your elders on financial issues. Don't hesitate to ask! The more proactive about financial planning your elders (and you!) are now, the more prepared everyone will be for the future—unexpected emergencies and all.

Resources on Financial Issues Relating to Elders

AARP (http://www.aarp.org/money/): Web page features information specifically about money matters related to elders.

Area Agency on Aging (AAA): Can be found in every state and often by county. Offers staff social workers and volunteers who can help facilitate discussions with elders and provide advice about how and when to establish financial control. Check out http://www.eldercarelocator.com to find the AAA in your community.

National Council on Aging (https://www.ncoa.org): Offers numerous resources for elders and their families on their website and provides links to local resources.

SmartAboutMoney.org: A National Endowment for Financial Education website that offers information about how to plan for yourself or for an elder's diminished capacity to handle money.

There's an App for That!

The following apps help you to organize your finances and categorize spending: **Mint, Spendee, Manilla, Slice**, and **Expensify**. They are available on iOS and Android. Search your app store for "organizing finances" for other similar apps.

GETTING ORGANIZED

So many steps, so many details, so little time! The bottom line of financial management is that you can't make a plan if you don't have all the specifics. Your elders need to know where their money currently comes from, where to find it, where it's going, and if they're going to have enough to last for the rest of their lives. The best way to do that is to have really good records.

Pulling records together takes time, though, so be patient with your elders and assist them in methodically documenting their accounts one step, one form, at a time.

To start the process, fill out the **"Getting Organized"** financial forms available for download at https://rowman.com/ISBN/9781442265462—and then keep all the filled-out forms together in a special binder.

One of the forms you will find is a "Collectibles Inventory" chart for recording coin and stamp collections, jewelry, and other collectibles.

While gathering the information, we recommend your elders also track down and compile the following important financial documents:

- Tax returns for the last five to seven years
- Documents related to asset purchases
- Insurance policies (home, auto, etc.)
- Statements of accounts (bank, 401K, investments, etc.)
- Deeds to house or condo, or other property
- Title transfers
- Car title and registration
- RV, boat, and other recreational vehicle titles and registrations
- Gifting information for estate tax purposes
- Military service records including years of service, branch, and identification numbers
- Wills and trust documents

Elder-Friendly Computers

If your elder can take advantage of the efficiencies of the Internet Age, then being able to use a computer will make collecting and storing all the valuable documents easier as well as allow you and your elder to access tons of valuable resources. To that end, throughout *Eldercare 101*, we feature Internet links to resources and online programs you will want to explore. To do so, you will want to know about the elder-friendly computers and tablets available on the market. Increasingly, developers are creating easy-to-use tablets or computers that are bundled with software, apps, and Wi-Fi capabilities. These products may be limited to the bundled software provided and can't necessarily be expanded to new apps and software. Many have larger print and recognizable icons that guide elders to the capabilities they most need in a computer or tablet. Many include the ability for relatives and friends to access the computer if the elder is having problems. Some include a monthly service program which enables the computer as a health-tracking system and emergency-alert system. The following are a few products, but this is a growing market, so do an online search for "computers for seniors [or elders]" and "tablets for seniors [or elders]" before you purchase one.

AARP RealPad: http://www.aarprealpad.org/
Claris Companion Tablet: http://clariscompanion.com/
InTouch Tablets: http://seniortouchpad.com/
Telikin Computers: http://telikin.com/

The Durable (Financial) Power of Attorney Representative

We also highly recommend that you suggest to your elders that they review their documents (and the forms they fill out) with their financial POA, at least one of their children, a trusted friend, or an ALCM. Elders will want to designate a POA and give someone they trust the authority to watch over their finances when they cannot or when they no longer want the burden. We cannot stress enough that asking for help is a very smart move, especially when it comes to money matters!

WHERE TO KEEP IMPORTANT DOCUMENTS

As noted in our "Legal" section, keeping important documents in a home safe, strongbox, or bank safe deposit box is a good protection from fire and theft. If your elders choose a bank safe deposit box or a lockbox in the home, be sure the DPOA representative knows the location of the key(s)—and inventory everything in the box.

> Forms for noting the details of where important documents are kept and how to access the location, as well as a **"Strong Box Inventory"** form, can be found at https://rowman.com/ISBN/9781442265462.

Note: If there is only one signature on file for the safe deposit box, add one or more signatures. Make sure this a trusted person or the person identified as the DPOA. This person should have access to the box in case of incapacity or death.

Digital Options

- **Flash Drive Storage:** Another way to stay organized, in addition to keeping copies of financial records and other important documents in a binder or in another central, safe place is to save all the information on a flash drive. You can scan important documents, the forms you print and fill out from https://rowman.com/ISBN/9781442265462, create a password-protected file, and save to a portable flash drive—or two! Keep one of the flash drives in an emergency preparedness kit and another safely locked away in a fireproof box or a safe deposit box.
- **Online Storage:** You can keep electronic documents safe, backed up, and accessible online from anywhere by storing them in the Cloud through

programs such as **Dropbox** (https://www.dropbox.com). Many other e-commerce companies—such as **AboutOne** (http://www.aboutone .com)—will organize and store financial information for you as well. Many such online services are free or charge a nominal fee.

To find a safe and secure option that's the right solution for your elders, ask for a referral from a trusted advisor. If you decide to locate an online service provider yourself, you can do an online search using the keywords: "secure personal information storage." Here also are some tips for making sure the option is safe:

- The provider should use firewalls, redundant hardware, redundant power sources, redundant battery backups, redundant cooling and redundant babbling, and video surveillance. You should find all this information on the provider's website.
- The provider should use encryption and software that tests the security of the provider.
- Information should be backed up regularly, and the backups should be encrypted.
- Look for identification of virus protection such as **McAfee** and **Norton**. Also, **TRUSTe** and **DigiCert** are companies that certify the privacy standards of providers. Look for their emblems.
- Only use trusted sources you have thoroughly vetted. You might even double check your choice or verify a company's standing through:
    Better Business Bureau: http://www.bbb.org
    DigiCert: https://www.digicert.com
    International Association of Privacy Professionals (IAPP): https:// www.iapp.org
    TRUSTe: http://www.truste.com

RETIREMENT INCOME

When elders are determining if they will have enough money to carry them through their end of life, the place to start is with income. Perhaps the elder for whom you care still works or works part time. Perhaps he collects a pension, lives off dividends and investment income, or receives Social Security benefits. Whatever the income, record and keep track of that income. Also, when the elder dies, knowing the source of the income and if any survivor benefits are available is helpful.

For tracking forms for **"Retirement Income,"** go to https://rowman.com/ISBN/ 9781442265462.

About Pensions

Elders often have government or private company pension benefits. These benefits are managed by a pension fund and are distributed directly from the administrator. The recipient does not usually control the investments, and *the benefits often end when the recipient dies*. The benefit plan may be a defined contribution plan or a defined benefit plan.

A defined contribution plan is a plan through which an employee can make contributions to his account with payroll deductions either before or after taxes. An employer also may make contributions to the plan. The account is generally tax deferred until withdrawals begin.

A defined benefit plan, also known as a traditional pension plan, promises the employee a specified monthly benefit at retirement. The amount is generally based on factors such as the employee's salary, age, and the number of years of service. The employee is not required to contribute to the plan. Taxes are paid when distributions begin.

Both plans are taxed the same and have similar benefits at death. You can contact the plan administrator directly for more information on pension benefits. If you are not the beneficiary or account owner of the plan, you will need the DPOA to access this information.

Understanding Social Security Benefits

If you have questions about Social Security benefits, you can request a **Benefit Verification Letter** online at http://www.ssa.gov. Or you can call 1-800-772-1213 (TTY 1-800-325-0778), Monday through Friday from 7 a.m. to 7 p.m. Note: If you are not the account holder, you will need a DPOA to transact any business on behalf of the elder.

The Benefit Verification Letter also is sometimes called a "budget letter," a "benefits letter," a "proof of income letter," or a "proof of award letter." It is an official letter from the Social Security Administration outlining current benefits and can be used as proof of:

- Income when applying for a loan or mortgage
- Income for assisted housing or other state or local benefits
- Current Medicare health insurance coverage

- Retirement status
- Disability
- Age

When you request a Benefit Verification Letter, you will be asked to select what information you want included or left out of the benefits letter. You also can set up an online account through http://www.ssa.gov/myaccount. This account can help your elder:

- Keep track of earnings and verify them every year
- Get an estimate of future benefits if she is still working
- Get a letter with proof of benefits if she currently receives them
- Manage benefits
  - ○ Change address
  - ○ Start or change direct deposit
  - ○ Get a replacement SSA-1099 or SSA-1042S for tax season

In addition, the benefits eligibility tool can be used to find out the benefits for which your elder might be eligible and learn how to qualify and apply as well. **The Benefits Eligibility Screening Tool (BEST) can be found online at** http://ssabest.benefits.gov/.

Social Security Death Benefits

When a spouse who has been receiving Social Security benefits passes away, the surviving spouse or DPOA should contact Social Security as soon as possible. As of 2016, a one-time death benefit of $255 is paid to the surviving spouse, or, if there is no surviving spouse, to the worker's child (or children) under certain circumstances. If the eligible surviving spouse is not currently receiving benefits, he or she must apply for this payment *within two years of the date of death*. For more information about this lump-sum payment, contact the local Social Security office or call 1-800-772-1213 (TTY 1-800-325-0778). Currently, the application is not available online.

To request Social Security death benefits, the following original documents will be required (in most states, photocopies are not accepted):

- Birth certificate or other proof of birth
- Proof of citizenship or lawful alien status
- U.S. military discharge papers
- W-2 forms or self-employment tax returns for last year
- Death certificate for the deceased

Social Security and Same-Sex Couples

Whereas many states are changing how benefits are determined for same-sex couples, Social Security is now processing some retirement, surviving spouse, and lump-sum death payment claims for same-sex couples in non-marital legal relationships and paying benefits that are due. If your elder is in such a relationship and his partner dies, your elder should apply right away for benefits, even if he isn't sure he is eligible. Applying quickly will protect surviving loved ones against the loss of any potential benefits. Also, the same-sex partner should apply for *retirement* benefits as soon as possible if the other partner is currently receiving Social Security benefits. The surviving partner should apply for the *death* benefits mentioned earlier within two years of the date of death.

Apply online at https://www.socialsecurity.gov for:

- Retirement or spouse's benefits
- Medicare benefits
- Disability benefits
- Extra help with Medicare prescription drug costs

Online application for Survivors Benefits is currently unavailable. Instead, contact the local Social Security office or call the national Social Security number at 1-800-772-1213 for that information. The following documents will be required for the application:

- Proof of death (either from the funeral home or death certificate)
- Social Security number of applicant and the Social Security number of the deceased
- Birth certificate of applicant
- Marriage certificate
- Proof of U.S. citizenship or lawful alien status
- Deceased worker's most recent W-2 forms or federal self-employment tax return
- Bank name and account number for applicant (so benefits can be directly deposited)

NOTES ON INDIVIDUAL RETIREMENT ACCOUNTS

Many elders contributed to individual retirement accounts (IRAs) or participated in other company-sponsored retirement plans during their working years. These accounts can be self-directed (invested directly by the participant) or directed by the sponsoring company and can include:

- **Traditional IRAs and Roth IRAs.** Retirement accounts that have been set up directly by the participant/employee subject to the contribution limits at the time of contribution. Generally made with post-tax dollars that may or may not have had a deduction on the federal tax return.
- **Rollover IRAs.** IRAs that were in a company-sponsored defined contribution plan that became the participant's at separation of service. Contributions are generally made with pre-tax dollars.
- **SIMPLE (Savings Incentive Match Plans for Employees) IRAs.** Allow employees and employers to contribute to traditional IRAs set up for employees. Contributions are generally made with pretax dollars.
- **SEP (Simplified Employee Pension) IRAs.** Allow employers to contribute to traditional IRAs set up for employees. Generally used by self-employed persons, and a deduction is generally available for the employer.
- **401(k) and 403(b) Plans.** Allow employees to contribute a portion of their wages to individual accounts generally on a pre-tax basis.

Other types of retirement plans that are not generally used have special rules regarding contributions and distributions such as Money Purchase Plans, Employee Stock Ownership Plans (ESOPs), 457 Plans, and Nonqualified Deferred Compensation Plans. If your elder has one of these, contact a tax advisor regarding the rules surrounding distributions, transfers, and taxation.

If you are not the beneficiary or account owner of one of these plans, you will need to have a DPOA to access information from the plan administrator.

Note #1: Taking MRDs

Generally, one has to take **Minimum Required Distributions (MRDs)** from any retirement account to which one contributed tax-deferred assets or had tax-deferred earnings. MRDs are mandatory, minimum yearly withdrawals that generally *must be taken starting in the year one turns age seventy and a half.* Whereas there is a minimum amount required to withdraw to avoid severe penalties, one can always take more than the MRD amount. Also, the majority of the accounts *can begin paying at age fifty-nine and a half* and continue until the recipient dies or the account runs out of money. Each account has very specific rules on how the money is distributed upon death.

Note #2: Designating Beneficiaries

Make sure your elder has determined or updated the beneficiaries on these accounts. A good rule of thumb is to review and update every two years. *Distri-*

butions from these accounts after death go directly to the stated beneficiaries regardless of what a will or living trust states. Consult with an attorney specializing in estates and elder law to determine the proper beneficiary designation.

Note #3: Inherited IRAs

Inherited IRAs have special rules for MRDs, and the required distributions are time sensitive, usually beginning in the year after the year of death of the original owner. Consult a professional financial advisor before distributing any money from an inherited IRA. You can find information on selecting a CPA in your area at the American Institute of Certified Public Accountants' website, http://www.aicpa.org. Your state also will have a society of CPAs you can contact for more information. See more information about finding the right CPA in our "Types of Financial Professionals" section toward the end of this chapter.

Note #4: Consolidating Retirement Accounts

Consider consolidating retirement accounts. Many of the plans listed previously can be rolled over into one or two accounts to make the management of them much easier. We recommend you speak with a CPA or investment professional about this strategy.

> For forms to facilitate documentation of **"Individual Retirement Accounts,"** go to https://rowman.com/ISBN/9781442265462.

TIPS FOR ELDERS ABOUT BANK ACCOUNTS

Tip #1: Appoint a DPOA Representative

You may be doing fine right now, paying bills on your own. But what happens if you become ill or incapacitated? As noted numerous times already in *Eldercare 101*—and repeated because of its importance—we recommend planning ahead and selecting a DPOA representative. Alternatively, you can hire a bill-paying service, which we'll talk about later in this section under "Getting Help with Bill Paying."

Tip #2: Close Accounts No Longer Being Used

While this may not be a good idea for younger people establishing credit, it can protect elders from fraud and simplify the financial picture.

Tip #3: Review Checkbooks and Bank Statements at Least Bimonthly

Pencil in two days on your calendar, perhaps the fifteenth and the thirtieth of each month, for a systematic review of accounts. Ask, "Does everything match up? Do the numbers make sense? Is there anything suspicious?" Pay careful attention to large transactions and transfers between accounts to make sure all money is accounted for.

Tip #4: Bank Online

Having access to your bank accounts online can save time—as well as trees! You can check balances, confirm transfers, and even pay bills online. If you do not have access to your accounts online, talk to your banker and investment advisors. Have them set up your accounts with a username and password and show you how to navigate the financial institution's website. Online banking also can be helpful when you are being assisted with bill paying by a caregiver or a child who does not live nearby.

There's an App for That!

Almost all banks have apps for banking needs including transferring money, depositing checks, and paying bills. Search for the bank name in the app store. Your personal banker will be happy to help you set up and teach you how to use the app.

Tip #5: Combine Accounts

The easiest way to simplify a financial life is to reduce the number of accounts you have. Generally, only one checking account and one savings account is needed to manage a household. The same goes for credit cards; it makes sense to consolidate and have one main credit card and perhaps one additional card, in case of an emergency. Make sure credit cards have fraud protection included.

Tip #6: Review How Your Accounts Are Held

- Joint or single?
- In trust or held individually?

- Determine who has authority to sign on the accounts. If necessary, update the signatures. This will require a trip to the bank with personal identification such as a driver's license, birth certificate, or passport.

Note these pitfalls of joint accounts: Once something is titled jointly, including checking and savings accounts, the account is truly joint. Either person can withdraw any amount at any time. *Also, when a person is deceased, all remaining funds go directly to the joint holder, regardless of direction in a will.* In addition, if the joint owner has credit issues or declares bankruptcy, the creditor can make a claim on the jointly owned account. Make sure the entire family is clear on this point before having a joint account.

Paid on Death (POD) may be a better option than a joint account. You can add a person to have authority to sign with a POA, but the account does not have to be a joint account. Unlike with the joint account, with the POD, you need to properly notify your bank whom you want to receive the account balance upon death. The bank may have a form to fill out and sign. Make sure you have proper identification when you talk to the banker about having an account POD. This type of beneficiary designation also will generally bypass probate upon death and is free. The beneficiary has no right to the money as long as the account owner is alive.

Tip #7: Ask If a Death Benefit Is Attached to the Account

Often, bank accounts will have a small death benefit as a perk for having the account. Inquire directly with the bank to see if a death benefit or small accidental life insurance is included with the account.

For **"Checking and Savings Accounts"** tracking forms, go to https://rowman. com/ISBN/9781442265462.

WHAT TO KNOW ABOUT INVESTMENTS

Most people own at least one or more different type of investments. An investment portfolio may be quite simple or very complicated. Even if you are not the primary financial decision maker, you need an understanding of what your elder's investments are and what the purposes are for the investments. Some investments are specifically purchased to generate cash flow; others are for short- or long-term savings goals. In addition, your financial and savings goals do and should change as you age. Reviewing investments at least annually is a good idea to see if your elders' investments still fit their financial goals. If they need help with this, please consult a personal investment advisor or a CFP®. Perhaps they'll want to compile and keep the investment statements in a special binder.

For detailed **"Investments"** tracking forms, go to https://rowman.com/ISBN/9781442265462.

Stocks

Your elders may have, or you may find, individual stock certificates. The easiest way to determine the value of these certificates or to sell them is to transfer them to a brokerage house (e.g., Fidelity, Vanguard, TD Ameritrade). The brokerage firm will then "hold" the certificates in an account for your elders. If they don't have a brokerage account, they can open one with a company that may hold other assets of theirs (i.e., retirement accounts). If needed, seek guidance from a financial investment advisor or CPA on how to manage this.

Bonds

Your elders may have, or you may find, individual bonds. Some of these may pay regular interest and some are worth more when cashed in at maturity. Consult a financial planner or investment advisor to determine what to do with individual bonds.

GIFT GIVING AND ESTATE PLANNING: IDEAS TO REVIEW WITH YOUR ELDER

If your elder has accumulated enough wealth that he may want to start gifting to children, grandchildren, or qualified charities, please contact an estate planner first. A qualified estate planner can help with a cash flow projection, look at the overall estate planning needs, and give good planning ideas for gifting while your elder is still alive. A gift from a warm hand is much better than a gift from a cold hand.

Many professionals can help with gift and estate planning. A CPA, financial advisor, bank trust officer, or attorney can get you started and offer planning ideas. Ask your planner how much experience he has had with similar situations, ask for referrals, and ask for a reasonable expectation of how much the planning will cost. Fees vary by professional and by the complexity of the gift and estate plan.

There are many ways to give gifts. Closely look at the desired outcome of the gift and your elder's personal tax situation. Here are a few ways to gift:

Gift Cash Outright

As of 2016, the annual gift exclusion per the Internal Revenue Service (IRS) is $14,000 per person to avoid a taxable gift. Each person is entitled to this exclusion. Together, two people can gift up to $28,000. This amount is inflation indexed and is released by the IRS generally in December each year.

Pay Tuition or Medical Expenses Directly

There is a gift tax exclusion for tuition or medical expenses paid directly on behalf of the recipient. The gift exclusion does not apply to these gifts. If you pay the medical facility or the qualified school directly the amount due (even if above $14,000), there is no taxable gift.

Gift Appreciated Securities

Appreciated securities are investments whose fair market value is greater than the cost of the security. The fair market value is used for the amount of the gift. For example, your elder has stock that is worth $14,000. He paid $1,000 for the stock. The stock has an appreciation of $13,000. If your elder gifts the stock to someone, the person has received a gift in the amount of $14,000. That person does not pay tax on the appreciation and neither does your elder. Current tax law says that the person receiving the stock has a "stepped-up" basis of $14,000. If the person sells the stock for $15,000, he will have a taxable gain of only $1,000. Again, talk with a professional advisor about these types of gifts.

Gift Giving to Divorced Children, Grandchildren, or Persons with Special Needs

There are a few things to consider when gifting to children who have been divorced, to grandchildren, or to persons with special needs. Your elder may need to consider gifting to a trust, a Section 529 plan for tuition, or other means of transferring the wealth. A Section 529 plan is a college education savings plan established by the IRS and operated by a state or an educational institution. Monies contributed to these plans generally grow tax-free as long as the contribution and investment earnings are used for education. For more information, check out http://www.savingforcollege.com, an excellent website for general information on these types of plans and the plans available in your state.

Tax Ramifications

Many states offer tax deductions for contributions to these plans as incentives for using their plan. Check with an estate professional for any deductions available for your elder's income tax return.

Making a gift or leaving an estate to heirs does not ordinarily affect federal income tax. Your elder cannot deduct the value of gifts made (other than gifts that are deductible charitable contributions or possibly state tax deductions for Section 529 plans). Gifts to charities are not subject to these limits and generally are tax deductible.

As of 2016, the federal estate tax exemption amount is $5,450,000 per person; it is currently inflation indexed every year. If you have a federal taxable estate, please contact an estate planning professional for useful planning ideas and tools.

Also, note that many states have different estate exemption amounts. To find out if your elder has a state taxable estate, please check with an estate planning professional in his area. Many states have estate planning councils that consist of attorneys, CPAs, trust officers, and other investment advisors. You can perform an Internet search for "estate planning council." These organizations can tell you what the local state exemption amount is.

Caregiver Tip Related to Monies Paid by You on Behalf of Your Elder

Monies paid by you on behalf of your elder may or may not be considered a gift. For example, medical expenses paid directly on behalf of another are excluded from being considered taxable gifts along with a few other exclusions. If you are paying more than the gift tax exclusion on behalf of your elder, please check with an attorney or other financial advisor to see if you have a taxable gift to report. As noted earlier, the federal gift tax exclusion for 2016 is $14,000 per person and is inflation adjusted each year.

BE SCAMWISE!

What is a scam? Individuals posing as fake businesses take advantage of people's trust, use pressure, threats, steal your money, and steal your identity. Scams can affect everyone—young, old, rich, poor, sophisticated, or naïve. Elders are especially targeted due to their acquired wealth, desire to help others, and lack of knowledge of current scams. Keep in mind that almost everyone has been scammed at some point in his life. Make sure your loved ones understand there is no need to be embarrassed if they have been the victims of a scam. Also, make sure the incident is reported.

Listed here are the most common scams. A phishing scam is hard to distinguish from a trusted source. Phishing scams are fake e-mails that look like the real e-mail you may receive from a trusted source. Scams look and sound like the real thing.

Fake mail from the Social Security Administration, IRS, or Medicare. The goal of this scam is to get you to provide information to steal your identity or access bank accounts. The Social Security Administration, IRS, and Medicare do *not* contact consumers through e-mail.

Phony fraud alerts. "There has been suspicious activity on your account." Real banks and financial institutions do not contact customers about fraud alerts via e-mail. Real banks and financial institutions do not ask for credit card information if they initiated the call. Use the phone number provided on your statement or on the back of your credit card to make inquiries.

Jury duty scams. A person will call to say, "You failed to report for jury duty and a warrant has been issued for your arrest." He will try to get a Social Security number. Courts do not use the phone or e-mail. They use U.S. mail.

Nigerian 419 scams and sweepstakes scams. This scam is designed to steal your account information or have you send money directly. This can be through e-mail, mail, or a phone call. If it is an e-mail, do not open the e-mail. Do not reply, even to unsubscribe. Just delete it.

Charity scams. These take advantage of your generosity and kindness. The goal is to steal your credit card information, as well as to get actual donations. These scams can be quite persuasive. Never make decisions about donations under pressure. If the charity is legitimate, the opportunity to donate will always be available.

Grandchild in trouble scams. A person will get an emotional phone call from someone claiming to be a relative. The scam artist is requesting money immediately and wants it wired to him. Every year thousands of unsuspecting grandparents lose money to grandchild scams.

Fake online pharmacies and Medicare scams. These scams offer very cheap prices for needed drugs without requiring a prescription from a doctor. Legitimate online pharmacies will require a valid prescription before they send out medications and will always have full contact details listed on their websites.

Investment seminar scams. These scams try to convince you to make investments that are either fake or not in your best interest. They usually include a free lunch and an expert who will give advice. The goal of the seminar is usually to schedule a private meeting in your home, where they pressure you to make a decision. Always get independent financial advice.

Opt-out negative option scams. Free thirty-day trial! When the trial is over, you are automatically charged for the item unless you cancel it within a specified time frame. Negative marketing is usually legal, so be very cautious of free trial offers. Review bank and credit card statements monthly and dispute charges quickly. *In most states, you only have fifty days to dispute charges.*

Construction and home repair scams. These scammers work door-to-door and offer to perform services or repairs for free or at a reduced price. Door-to-door solicitors and telemarketing calls offering home repair services should always be viewed as highly suspect. They may pretend to do work and charge for unnecessary repairs. Never pay for repairs upfront! Wait until the work is completed.

The best way to protect elders from scams is through education. Once you recognize a scam, you need to know how to resist the pitch. Just say, "No"! Being scammed is nothing to be ashamed of. One of the reasons scam artists are successful is because people are reluctant to report being scammed. Reporting scams is the only way regulatory agencies can monitor trends.

First Rule of Being Scamwise?

Do not open, but delete, an e-mail if you are unsure who sent it to you is valid and/or you do not know the sender. If someone you know or someone with whom you do business wants to contact you, he will have your phone number. You also can check out http://www.Snopes.com to check if the e-mail is a valid request or a scam.

What to Do If You Have Been the Victim of a Scam?

Contact the attorney general's office of your state. To locate the attorney general for your state, go to http://www.naag.org/.

How Do I Place a Fraud Alert/Security Freeze on My Credit Report?

You may call any one of the credit bureaus or request a fraud alert or security freeze online. You also may contact the other two bureaus if you wish, but fraud alerts are shared with the other bureaus once you place one with a single bureau.

General Resources on Scams

http://www.aarp.org/money/scams-fraud/
http://www.Snopes.com
http://www.scamwatch.gov.au

Resources on Unsolicited Mail, Telemarketing, and E-mail Fraud

https://www.donotcall.gov or call 1-888-382-1222
https://www.dmachoice.org/index.php
Call 1-888-567-8688 to opt out of preapproved credit offers.

Charity Fraud Resources

BBB Wise Giving Alliance: http://www.give.org
American Institute of Philanthropy: https://www.charitywatch.org
Charity Navigator: http://www.charitynavigator.org

PAYING THE BILLS

How do your elders handle the day-to-day and month-by-month demands of keeping up with bills? Do they have a bill-paying process in place? Are they diligent about paying credit card bills on time so as not to incur interest charges? If they still own their home, are they up to date on their mortgage payments so they are not paying penalties? Is the sheer volume of bills overwhelming them? Are they concerned they can no longer take care of paying recurring bills?

We will delve into specific aspects of bill paying in the rest of this section, however, to get started, here are some easy steps we encourage your elders to put in place right away:

- **Establish and commit to keeping track of spending habits.** Many elders may simply use a check register to track their cash balance and may not be aware of how they are spending their money. Tracking spending as people age becomes more and more important because resources may become less while costs continue to climb.
- **Keep track of deadlines and due dates.**
- **Sort through mail daily.** Look for credit card statements, bank statements, requests for money, and other invoices. Make sure everything matches up with your knowledge of the spending. If something is wrong, act quickly to investigate.
- If you haven't already done so, **establish online bank accounts**.
- **Set up direct deposit of checks and automatic payment of recurring bills.**
- **Shred all discarded documents.**

CREDIT AND DEBIT CARD TIPS FOR ELDERS

Your wallet or purse can be a great place to start in getting your bills under control.

Tip #1: Record Information

Pull out all your credit and debit cards, and document each card as you handle it. Look for the contact phone numbers on the back of the cards.

One strategy for documenting them is to record all the information on the **"Credit and Debit Card Accounts"** form available at https://rowman.com/ISBN/9781442265462.

Otherwise, you might take photos of the debit cards with your smartphone or camera so you can refer to the information as needed or in the event of theft. Once you print the photos and store the photos in a safe place, you can delete them from your mobile device.

Tip #2: Live Simply

Regarding credit cards, once you get a sense of all you have, you may want to consider closing most of the accounts and utilizing only one or two—one you mostly use, and one to have as a backup. Having fewer credit cards really simplifies your financial picture!

Tip #3: Safeguard the Cards

When carrying credit cards on your person or while traveling, use an aluminum/metal wallet so credit card information cannot be stolen by passersby with high-tech scamming devices.

RECURRING PAYMENTS

If your elders still own their home, consider the routine: Every month they have bills for electricity, heat, garbage pickup, water usage, homeowner's insurance, maybe a lawn service, and more. Maybe they tithe to their place of worship monthly, or pay a housecleaner the same amount weekly. These charges are "recurring," which means they recur weekly, monthly, bimonthly, quarterly, or annually. Even if your elders don't own their home, they might have recurring charges for insurance, an assisted living facility, or an adult foster home.

Automate the Recurring Payments . . .

Whatever the recurring charge, it pays to automate! Most companies allow for automatic payment of recurring charges via bank accounts or as a credit card charge. Setting up the automatic payments can be time consuming at first, but, in the long term, doing so will save tons of time in personal bill paying. For bills that are not the same amount every month, check with the provider to see if the fees can be "evened out" throughout the year so your elder has predictability in how his checking account or credit card bill is affected. Many utilities offer this option.

Note: There are certain types of payments that should never be automated—such as for credit card(s)! These you want to be sure to watch closely on a regular basis and pay separately.

. . . and Track Them!

Understanding recurring charges is also a great place to start when establishing—and sticking to—a budget. Sit down with your elder and encourage him to take the time to record the dates, amounts, and payees of his recurring payments. For example, does he pay insurance fees online or through an automatic bank charge or on his credit card? If so, which bank account or credit card? How much is automatically deducted or charged? What day of the month is the fee deducted or charged? Tracking recurring payments now will help you or a service assist with bill paying, if your elder ever needs help. **Quicken software**, **Quicken.com**, and **Mint.com** are all useful tools for tracking spending.

> For a **"Recurring Payments"** form, go to https://rowman.com/ISBN/ 9781442265462.

BILL-PAYING STRATEGIES

Setting good bill-paying habits now and getting the help needed will ensure that, as your elders age, they will be more comfortable managing their finances and having a plan in place to have their finances managed by someone else when they can no longer do it. Elders have a variety of options for getting help. They can:

- Ask a trusted loved one or friend to take over *just* bill paying.
- Appoint a trusted person to be their DPOA.
- Hire a conservator to take over their complete financial management, when needed.

If your elder doesn't have anyone willing or able to personally help, professional help is available. Check in your area for:

- **Bank Trust Officers and Elder Lawyers:** These professionals can assist with setting up trusts and other bill-paying services.
- **CPAs:** CPAs are a good option, if your elder also needs assistance preparing tax returns.
- **Aging Life Care Managers:** The Aging Life Care Association (http://www.aginglifecare.org) is a nonprofit organization that provides referrals for licensed professionals who work with older adults and their adult children and loved ones to develop holistic aging plans and programs addressing all aspects of aging. About 20 percent of ALCMs also provide daily money management services.
- **Daily Money Manager (DMM) Bill-Paying Services:** These programs can be offered through a nonprofit or a for-profit agency. They help people who cannot handle their own financial affairs by assisting with bill paying, balancing checkbooks, reviewing statements, and maintaining records. In essence, representatives of the DMM act as personal financial assistants. Their services are normally billed by the hour and can vary by region. If your elder is considering using a DMM, be sure he compares fees, checks references, verifies agencies, and ensures that the individual or company is bonded. In fact, you should always use extra caution when selecting anyone who will have access to your finances! Your elder also should always retain or give *only* to his POA check-signing responsibilities. The potential for fraud should not be overlooked, and neither federal nor state governments currently regulate the DMM industry.

To Find a DMM

The best way to start your search is through referrals, the American Association of Daily Money Managers (AADMM) at http://www.aadmm.com, and your local elder assistance agencies. To find elder assistance agencies in your area, contact your local Area Agency on Aging. The federal government's website at http://www.eldercare.gov will have your local information. During your research, you may find some local government agencies that offer free services through volunteers or provide referrals to other nonprofits that may provide assistance.

Important questions to ask potential DMMs either by phone interview or in person:

- What services do they provide?
- How do they charge and what is their rate?
- Do they charge for other fees such as travel time, office supplies, or postage?
- What type of training have they had?

- How long have they been working as a DMM?
- What type and how much insurance do they have?
- Are they bonded?
- Are they certified as a professional DMM?
- Ask for references!

GETTING A CREDIT REPORT

Are you certain your elder's credit is good? Concerned someone might have stolen his identity? Want to be sure he will be approved for a loan? Did his partner manage their finances for years and now you want a sense of where your elder stands financially? A credit report can provide all the answers.

Every person is entitled to one free credit report per year. Start with https://www.annualcreditreport.com or order online from any of the following credit bureaus:

Experian: http://www.experian.com
Equifax: http://www.equifax.com
Transunion: http://www.transunion.com

Warning: Be careful of the pop-up ads when completing online orders. You do *not* need to pay or enter credit card information to have access to the reports, but you are required to enter personal information and provide an e-mail address.

Once You Have the Report? Be Sure to Review for Accuracy!

You don't know what you don't know. Dispute any inaccurate information. As a consumer, you have a right to dispute any item you feel is incorrect on your credit report. To dispute an item, you would follow the dispute process of the particular credit bureau you used; all three bureaus have an online dispute process. You need to go to each reporting bureau to dispute the item. The bureaus do not share this information.

More about Credit Reports and Credit Issues

Basic Information about Credit

http://www.consumer.ftc.gov/articles/0155-free-credit-reports
http://www.consumerfinance.gov/askcfpb/search?q=credit

Credit Reports and Scores

http://www.consumer.ftc.gov/articles/0152-how-credit-scores-affect-price-
   credit-and-insurance
http://www.consumerfinance.gov/askcfpb/search?selected_facets=category_
   exact:credit-reporting

Your Right to a Free Report

http://www.consumer.ftc.gov/articles/0155-free-credit-reports/
http://www.consumerfinance.gov/askcfpb/search?selected_facets=tag
   _exact%3Afree+credit+report

Building a Better Report and Repairing Your Credit

http://www.consumer.ftc.gov/articles/0155-free-credit-reports/
http://www.consumerfinance.gov/askcfpb/318/how-do-i-get-and-keep-a-
   good-credit-score.html

Protecting against Fraud and Identify Theft

http://www.consumer.ftc.gov/features/feature-0014-identity-theft
http://www.consumerfinance.gov/askcfpb/search?selected_facets=tag_
   exact%3Aidentity+theft

THE FIRST THREE STEPS OF WHAT TO DO ABOUT DEBT

Have you discovered your elder has debt issues? Can he not afford the mortgage? Have credit card balances grown? For people living on fixed incomes, escalating debt can lead to financial ruin. You'll want to make getting your elder's debts under control a priority. You may want to encourage your elder to seek advice initially from a professional advisor. CFP®s and estate attorneys have special training in this area and can help you and your elder get started in resolving the problems. If your elder has an accountant or an attorney, have him schedule an appointment to discuss the debt burden. You also can get advice from the Consumer Credit Counseling Services (CCCS) at http://credit.org/cccs. All CCCS agencies are nonprofit organizations.

Step #1: Document Your Debt

For **"Debt Documentation"** forms, go to https://rowman.com/ISBN/
9781442265462.

Step #2: Get Credit Counseling Help

The National Foundation for Credit Counseling (http://www.nfcc.org) is a nonprofit counseling organization. The organization's website has valuable information and can point you to resources in your area. Once you find the right resource, schedule a meeting and take a list of your elder's debt issues with you.

Step #3: Try Some Debt-Management Strategies

Brainstorm with a credit counselor about debt-management strategies that can help reduce debt burden. For example, if your elder is still living at home, he has a valuable asset. In fact, his home can be tapped in many ways to provide for his care or debt reduction. Here are some suggestions for consideration:

- House share. You may know someone you trust who is willing and able to pay rent.
- Rent out the current home and move to a smaller home, apartment, or other housing option.
- Sell the current home and downsize to a smaller house or apartment. If your elder has an in-home caregiver, check with an ALCM for advice before selling the home. *There are options within special rules for the transfer of a home when you have a caregiver living in your home for two or more years.*
- Get a reverse mortgage if the current home is fully paid. Always talk to one or more financial management professionals about this choice, because a reverse mortgage has many pros and cons.

Pros of Reverse Mortgages

- Allow people sixty-two or older to convert home equity into cash without having to move or assume extra debt.
- The cash is received on a monthly basis, in a one-time lump sum payment, or as a credit line to use whenever needed.
- The money received from a reverse mortgage doesn't need to be paid back—as long as the owner continues to live in the house.
- May create a source of income that could last the rest of the elder's life.

Cons of Reverse Mortgages

- Must be repaid upon the homeowner's death. This can be paid by the estate of the deceased or the heirs of the deceased. Reverse mortgage lenders often give heirs from three to twelve months to repay the loan in full. If neither the estate nor the heirs repay the loan, the lender typically repossesses the home.

- The house will not be left to any heirs.
- Annual certification that the homeowner is in the house and that taxes and insurance are being paid is required.
- The transaction costs of obtaining a reverse mortgage are very high. Pay close attention to the fees. Often these fees are deducted from the equity in the home, reducing the net amount to the homeowner.
- The rules are very complicated. Again, check with a trusted advisor before agreeing to a reverse mortgage.

UNDERSTANDING THE COST OF CARE

If your elder is in debt and looking for some debt-management strategies, you may be hoping to leverage his home for some financial relief. Before doing anything, however, there are many questions to ask! How much really will your elder save by moving to an apartment, an assisted living facility, an adult foster home, or another housing option? Even if he isn't in debt, if he is still living at home and paying for any type of home care, the costs can quickly add up—and it would be prudent to compare the costs of staying in the home versus moving. Working through these issues with a financial advisor can prevent costly mistakes. An ALCM also can help with evaluating costs of staying in a home as compared to moving to an assisted living facility.

> For a **"Cost of Care"** worksheet, go to https://rowman.com/ISBN/
> 9781442265462.

Ready Resource

If your elder is considering a nursing home or anticipates needing home health care, the Medicare website http://www.medicare.gov/nursinghome compare/search.html is an excellent resource for comparing nursing homes, learning about long-term care options, and comparing other providers and home health care.

> **There's an App for That!**
>
> For average pricing of assisted care facilities and in-home care services in your area, also check out the **Genworth Cost of Care app**, https://www.genworth. com/corporate/about-genworth/industry-expertise/cost-of-care.html.

INSURANCE

Before your head starts spinning, insurance can be a valuable tool to help with money matters—once you understand the purpose and function of each type of insurance. In this section, we will highlight the various features of each of the following types:

- Medical and Health
- Homeowner's and Renter's
- Auto
- Life (including Term Life, Universal Life, and Whole Life)
- Veterans
- Liability/Umbrella
- Disability
- Long-Term Care (LTC)

As we explore insurances with you, we highly recommend you help your elders document all the types of insurance they have. Listing all their policies in one place can alleviate some of the "overwhelm" they might feel when thinking about insurance and being prepared for the future.

For a **"Documentation of Insurances"** form, go to https://rowman.com/ ISBN/9781442265462.

TYPES OF INSURANCES

Medicare and Private Pay Supplemental Health Insurance

Medical insurance can be provided through private pay or the government. The federally funded health insurance for people who are sixty-five or older (and younger people with certain disabilities) is **Medicare**. The website https://www.medicare.gov has valuable information on options, agencies to contact, and how to change coverage. **Medicare Part A (hospital insurance)** covers inpatient hospital stays, care in a skilled nursing facility, hospice care, and some home health care. **Medicare Part B (medical insurance)** covers certain doctors' services, outpatient care, medical supplies, and preventive services. Other parts of Medicare are supplemented through private companies under various programs, discussed next.

Medicare Advantage Plans (Medicare Part C)

These are a type of Medicare health plan offered by a private company that contracts with Medicare to provide all Part A and Part B benefits. If your elder is enrolled in a Medicare Advantage Plan, Medicare services are covered through the plan and aren't paid for under Original Medicare. Most Medicare Advantage Plans offer prescription drug coverage. Types of Medicare Advantage Plans include:

- **Health Maintenance Organization (HMO) Plans:** In most HMOs, the patient can only go to doctors, other healthcare providers, or hospitals in the plan's network except in an urgent or emergency situation. Your elder also may need to get a referral from his primary care provider for tests or to see other doctors or specialists.
- **HMO Point-of-Service (HMOPOS) Plans:** These are HMO plans that may allow some services out-of-network for a higher copayment or coinsurance.
- **Preferred Provider Organization (PPO) Plans:** In a PPO, the patient pays less if he uses doctors, hospitals, and other healthcare providers who belong to the plan's network. The patient usually pays more if using doctors, hospitals, and providers outside the network.
- **Private Fee-for-Service (PFFS) Plans:** PFFS plans are similar to original Medicare in that the patient can generally go to any doctor, other healthcare provider, or hospital as long as he agrees to treat the patient. The plan determines how much it will pay doctors, other healthcare providers, and hospitals, and how much to pay when the patient gets care.
- **Special Needs Plans (SNPs):** SNPs provide focused and specialized health care for specific groups of people such as those who have both Medicare and Medicaid, live in a nursing home, or have certain chronic medical conditions.

Medicare Supplement (Medigap) Insurance

Medigap is sold by private companies and can help pay some of the healthcare costs that Medicare doesn't cover such as copayments, coinsurance, and deductibles. A Medigap policy is different from a Medicare Advantage Plan. Those plans are ways to get Medicare benefits, whereas a Medigap policy only supplements the Original Medicare benefits. A Medigap policy can be purchased from any insurance company that's licensed in your state to sell one. You can search the Medicare website for a policy in your area by going to http://www.medicare.gov/find-a-plan/questions/medigap-home.aspx.

Medicare Part D: Prescription Drug Coverage

Medicare Part D adds prescription drug coverage to Original Medicare, some Medicare Cost Plans, some Medicare PFFS Plans, and Medicare Medical

Savings Account Plans. These plans are offered by insurance companies and other private companies approved by Medicare. Medicare Advantage Plans also may offer prescription drug coverage that follows the same rules as Medicare Prescription Drug Plans.

Medicaid

Medicaid—the "Gold Plastic Card"—provides free or low-cost health coverage for people under the federal poverty level as well as individuals under the age of sixty-five who have disabilities and are otherwise not insurable; the latter is called having Disability Insurance Benefits (DIB). Under Medicaid, there are no deductibles or copayments. Medicaid also pays for prescription drugs and extended nursing home stays as well as residential services.

Medicaid is run jointly by the federal and state governments and, as noted earlier, is a need-based program. Details, costs, and coverage vary somewhat between states.

The federal healthcare marketplace at https://www.healthcare.gov has information on eligibility, how to apply, and your state's coverage. In general, states set individual eligibility criteria based on the federal poverty level and the amount of assets available to pay for health care. To be eligible, you also must satisfy residency requirements, immigration status, and documentation of U.S. citizenship.

Five-Year Medicaid Spend Down

Even if income exceeds Medicaid levels in your state, your elder may be eligible under Medicaid "spend down" rules. Under the "spend down" process, some states allow eligibility for Medicaid as "medically needy" even if your elder has too much income to qualify. Nonetheless, be warned that Medicaid rules vary from state to state and the rules change frequently.

Get Advice!

If you are faced with providing long-term care for an elder, it is critical you *get advice about proper planning on how to receive Medicaid benefits before acting on disposing of financial or personal assets*. A professional, such as an elder law attorney, can keep you from breaking some of the stringent divestiture rules, including the five-year look-back at transfers or gifts of assets.

Tip: Although it can be difficult to qualify for Medicaid, consult an elder law attorney to find out options, especially if there is a spouse involved. There are tools that can protect the spouse from impoverishment. For more on elder law attorneys and how they can help, see the "Legal" section of *Eldercare 101*.

Medical and Health Insurance Resources

There are free services available to help navigate health insurance options. Contact your elder's state's Senior Health Insurance Benefits Assistance (SHIBA or SHIP) program for free help from trained volunteers. Start with the Centers for Medicare and Medicaid Services website at https://www.cms. gov. This site will provide a link to your specific state. Alternatively, you can search online for "senior health insurance benefits assistance [your elder's state]." Every state has free assistance available. Examples of state SHIBA programs can be found at http://www.insurance.wa.gov/ and http://www. oregon.gov/dcbs/insurance/shiba/Pages/shiba.aspx.

Medical Savings Account (MSA) Plans

These plans combine a high-deductible health plan with a bank account. Medicare deposits money into the account (usually less than the deductible). The money can be used to pay for healthcare services during the year. MSA plans don't offer Medicare drug coverage. For drug coverage, your elder can join a Medicare Prescription Drug Plan. For more information about MSAs, visit https://www.medicare.gov/publications to view the booklet "Your Guide to Medicare Medical Savings Account Plans." You also can call 1-800-MEDICARE (1-800-633-4227) to ask if a copy can be mailed to you. TTY users should call 1-877-486-2048.

   Tip: It can be challenging to navigate the medical and health insurance maze of coverage and options. An ALCM can help guide you through the maze.

Homeowner's or Renter's Insurance

Purchasing homeowner's or renter's insurance can be done from most major insurance carriers. Pick at least three insurance companies to compare. Get a good understanding of:

• The amount of the deductible and the annual premium
• Types of claims covered
• Length of time it takes a claim to be paid
• The reputation of the company
• Do they have a physical office and a designated agent for you?

The Insurance Information Institute has an online tool called "Know Your Stuff" (https://www.knowyourstuff.org) that can help to guide you through a home inventory for estimating how much coverage will be needed.

Homeowner's and renter's insurance provides protection for belongings. Help your elders review their coverage, deductibles, discounts available, replacement coverage, and any special coverage they may need. Typically, computers, cameras, jewelry, art, antiques, musical instruments, and stamp or coin collections require additional coverage.

Homeowner's or renter's insurance needs can and do change over time. Do not forget to check on coverage for storage units. Some homeowner's policies cover storage units and some do not. Check to see if there is a dollar limit on the amount covered for storage units.

Tip: Your elder may be paying for coverage no longer needed. It may be time to do a thorough review of the coverage provided. In helping your elders with their review, make sure they understand whether they have cash value or replacement cost coverage, and whether or not the values are accurate for what they currently own.

Auto Insurance

Auto insurance protects against financial loss if there is an accident. The contract defines what is covered based on the premium payments. Auto insurance provides property, liability, and medical coverage. If your elder is no longer driving, contact the insurance company to see if coverage can be reduced. If your elder is still driving, should he be? Consult with an ALCM to begin the discussion about when to give up the keys. For more on driving as an elder, see "Transportation Issues" in our "Social" section.

Life Insurance

Life insurance is a contract with an insurance company that provides a lump-sum payment, known as a death benefit, to beneficiaries in the event of the insured's death in exchange for premiums (payments). If your elder owns life insurance, the first step is to determine what type of insurance it is. In general, there are three types of life insurance:

1. **Term Life Insurance:** Term life insurance is designed to provide financial protection for a specified time, such as ten, twenty, or thirty years. Premiums are level and guaranteed for that period. After the initial term ends, companies may offer continued coverage, usually at a substantially higher premium rate. Term life insurance is paid upon death in a lump sum. Term life insurance should not be considered an investment; it is a safety net for beneficiaries.

2. **Universal Life Insurance:** Universal life insurance is a type of permanent life insurance designed to provide lifetime coverage. Universal life insurance policies are flexible and may allow you to raise or lower premiums or coverage amounts during the lifetime of the covered person. Some universal life insurance products focus on providing both a death benefit and generating a cash value. This buildup of cash value is tax-deferred wealth accumulation. These types of policies generally have an investment option for the cash value in the policy. If your elder's policy has a cash value amount, it may be withdrawn to assist with paying bills and medical expenses. Consult a tax professional (CPA) before doing this to make sure the tax consequences have been addressed.

3. **Whole Life Insurance:** Whole life insurance is a permanent life insurance designed to provide lifetime coverage. Policy premiums are typically fixed, and, unlike term life insurance, whole life insurance has a cash value, which functions as a savings component and may accumulate tax-deferred over time. Whole life can be used as an estate planning tool to help preserve wealth for beneficiaries.

Tip: Death benefits from all types of life insurance are generally income tax-free.

Veteran's Insurance

In addition to the veteran's pension, veterans also may qualify for assistance with activities of daily living (ADLs). For example, assistance is available for veterans who have served at least one day (of their required ninety-day minimum) during a time of war and need help with ADLs. The Aid and Attendance and Housebound Improved Pension benefit, known as A&A, can cover the costs of caregivers in the home (including sons and daughters who are paid to be caregivers) or be used for assisted living or a nursing home.

The nonprofit website http://www.VeteranAid.org has great information on who qualifies and how you apply. The Veterans Administration has many resources available for veterans and family members. Go to http://www.benefits.va.gov/insurance/ for more information and locations in your area. Additional state and local resources are available through state Veterans Affairs (VA) offices, http://www.va.gov/statedva.htm, and Veterans Service Organizations at http://www1.va.gov/vso/index.asp.

Warning: Be aware of scams offering to help complete VA applications. If help is needed, contact a veterans' benefits coordinator in your area or ask an ALCM for assistance.

Liability/Umbrella Insurance

Umbrella insurance is extra liability insurance designed to help protect against major claims and lawsuits. It does this by providing additional liability coverage above the limits of the homeowner's, auto, and boat insurance policies. Umbrella insurance provides coverage for:

• Injuries
• Damage to property
• Certain lawsuits
• Slander, libel, false arrest, shock/mental anguish

Tip: If liability/umbrella insurance is already in place, think twice before canceling it. Make sure you are aware of your potential for liability.

Disability Insurance

Is your elder receiving disability insurance from either Social Security or through private pay? This type of insurance is usually paid when a person can no longer perform the duties of his job. Social Security Disability Insurance (SSDI) provides a floor beneath all other forms of disability insurance. As a safety net, it catches everyone who was either uninsured or underinsured. Contact the provider of the disability payment for an understanding of what the disability payment represents and how long the insurance is required to pay.

Long-Term Care Insurance

Long-term care (LTC) insurance helps provide for the cost of long-term care up to a predetermined benefit amount or duration. It provides assistance when a person needs help with ADLs. Policies vary regarding the amount of coverage, when the coverage begins, and when benefits are triggered. Benefits are generally available when a person needs help with at least two or three ADLs such as bathing, eating, dressing, using the toilet, walking, and cognitive impairment such as dementia or Alzheimer's disease. The Department of Health and Human Services Administration on Aging website at http://www.longtermcare. gov has a complete list of ADLs along with important facts to consider for purchasing LTC insurance or self-insuring for long-term care needs.

Depending on the policy, LTC insurance can be provided and coverage paid directly to:

• Nursing homes
• Assisted living facilities

- Adult daycare services
- Home care
- Home modification
- Care coordination

Most LTC insurance policies are based on a concept that gives an individual access to a pool of money in exchange for payment of monthly premiums over the years of their (usually working) lives. Insurance companies use complex formulas to determine how many people will need the insurance, how much it pays out, and how much they will earn on interest from premiums.

If your elder already has LTC insurance, great! If not, it may or may not make sense for him. Many factors should be considered in determining whether or not LTC insurance is a good investment. Age, current health, family history, and availability of other financial resources must be considered. In fact, given the "game" of insurance, it is wise to consider four major factors when thinking about purchasing LTC insurance:

1. **Benefit Period:** The length of time after a claim is filed and the insurer will pay for the care that will be provided or has been provided.
2. **Elimination Period of Deductible:** The length of time and the amount of money that must be paid out of pocket before the insurer starts to pay.
3. **Daily Benefit:** The maximum dollar amount the insurer will pay for care each day.
4. **Level of Inflation Protection:** The amount benefits will increase over time to keep up with the rising costs of inflation.

Ask for Help!

Because of its complexity, consult an objective professional for advice before purchasing LTC insurance. Your financial advisor, CFP®, CPA, or other noncommissioned investment advisor can review the pros and cons for your particular situation. If your elder already has LTC insurance, have him ask the agent who sold him the policy to review any exclusions, waiting periods, coverage limitations, and inflation adjustments. You also can check out the website of the American Association of Long-Term Care Insurance at http://www.aaltci.org for rate and care comparisons.

GETTING HELP WITH FINANCIAL PLANNING AND ADVICE

Of course, no one can be an expert in everything. If you need help with money matters, then seek the right advice from the right professional. Some professionals are experts at guiding, managing, and directing your financial assets; others are better at tax, cash flow, and planning advice. Let us explore the different types of money advisors and what they can and cannot do for you.

For a form to record the names and contact information of members of your elder's **"Financial Aging Life Care Team,"** go to https://rowman.com/ISBN/9781442265462.

TYPES OF FINANCIAL PROFESSIONALS

Many different professionals can help with financial planning and advice. The four basic types of financial professionals are:

• Accountants
• Financial Planners
• Investment Advisors
• Stockbrokers

To determine which advisor best fits your needs can be confusing. People also can call themselves a "financial advisor" without having any specialized education, training, or expertise. Some other common "titles" include: financial analyst, financial consultant, investment consultant, or wealth manager. These are generic titles and may be used by investment professionals who may or may not hold any specific designation. Ask your selected advisor for credentials and be sure you have an understanding of his fee structure. Also, we highly recommend consolidating financial accounts! There is no need to have multiple brokerage accounts and financial advisors. All stocks, bonds, and mutual funds can be held by the same institution once the appropriate advisor is selected.

Certified Public Accountants

What can a CPA do for you? A CPA cannot only help you with planning and filing for your taxes but also with cash management and budgeting, with ideas to help you save money, and with objective advice about alternate scenarios presented to you with respect to cash flow projections. To learn more about what a CPA can do for you, or to find one, check out the AICPA's website at http://www.aicpa.org/FORTHEPUBLIC/FINDACPA/Pages/FindACPA.aspx. Once you have identified a few CPAs in your area, check them out to make sure you pick one who is a good fit for you and your elder. Here are some questions to ask either over the phone or during an initial consultation:

- Does he have expertise working with your issue (e.g., inherited IRAs)?
- How many years of individual tax experience does he have?
- What licenses does he have? (For inherited IRAs, a CPA is needed.)
- Does he have an advanced degree?
- Will he represent your elder if audited?
- Will he review past tax returns at no charge?
- What fees will he charge and how does he charge?
- Is there anything you personally can do to keep the fees down?
- Most importantly, do you and your elder feel comfortable working with this person?

Financial Planners

Financial planners help individuals meet their short- and long-term financial goals by evaluating each client's current financial status and developing a program to meet his objectives. A person does not need any specialized training or licensing to be called a financial planner, but many financial planners do hold credentials that attest to their experience and education. For example, Certified Financial Planners™, also known as CFP®s:

- Have successfully passed extensive exams on asset protection planning, taxes, insurance, estate planning, and retirement.
- Are required to maintain their certifications by completing yearly continuing education programs.
- Have fiduciary responsibility to clients. (The CFP Board's Standards of Professional Conduct states: "A certificant shall at all times place the interest of the client ahead of his own. When the certificant provides financial planning or material elements of financial planning, the certificant owes the client the duty of care of a fiduciary as defined by the CFP Board.")

A CFP® may charge for services by fee or by commission. A fee-only CFP® may charge an hourly fee, flat fee, or percentage of your assets or income. A fee-only CFP® does not receive commission on products sold. A commission-only CFP® earns a commission on the sale of certain products. Note: This payment structure may create a conflict of interest, because the CFP® may suggest a product with a better commission that is not the best product for your elder.

To find a CFP® in your area, contact the Financial Planning Association at http://www.letsmakeaplan.org or the National Association of Personal Financial Advisors at http://www.napfa.org.

Investment Advisors

Investment advisors, also known as investment advisor representatives (IARs), provide advice regarding and management of securities. IARs must pass qualifying exams and must act with "an affirmative duty of 'utmost good faith and full and fair disclosure of all material fact,' as well as an affirmative obligation 'to employ reasonable care to avoid misleading' clients." According to the U.S. Supreme Court, IARs must be registered with the Security and Exchange Commission (SEC) and/or state securities regulator, depending on the value of the client assets under management. Note: Registered IARs also can be called asset managers, investment counselors, investment managers, portfolio managers, and wealth managers. Investment advisors must disclose how they are paid, which may be via one of several methods:

- **Hourly fee:** This may or may not be advantageous to your elder, and very few investment advisors charge in this manner. They will keep track of how much time they spend managing your elder's account including conducting trades, discussions regarding investment selection, time spent researching investment options, and so on. They will either invoice directly or deduct it directly from the account they manage on your elder's behalf.
- **Fixed fee:** Investment advisors may use this method if the consumer also participates in the management of his investments. They may provide advice or guidance on a quarterly, semi-annually, or annual basis for a set amount each year while the consumer performs the transactions. If you or your elder are comfortable completing the transaction yourself, this could save money in fees. However, this may not be a good option for investors who are not savvy.
- **Commission on the products they sell** (if he is also a broker). Commission-only advisors will only make money on products they sell. If your elder only needs asset allocation, stock, bond, or mutual fund advice, this may not be the right method. Your elder may end up with an advisor changing his investments to generate more commissions.
- **Percentage of the value of the assets they manage for you, sometimes called "fee only":** The advisor will charge a fee generally based on the assets under management (AUM). The percentage can be anywhere from 0.5 percent up to 5 percent of your total assets. However, because the advisor is only getting paid based on the dollar amount of AUM, he will most likely be acting in your elder's best interest.
- **A combination of the above methods.**

Many experts say that a fee-only advisor is preferable so as to eliminate conflict of interest and to ensure he always acts with your elder's best interests at heart. However, if your elder needs help with annuities or insurance products, he may need to go with a fee-only plus commissions. An investment advisor must be a broker-dealer to sell insurance products, and these are sold on commission. Typically, broker-dealers will use a combination of the discussed methods.

Stockbrokers

Stockbrokers are regulated professionals who make stock trades in exchange for a fee or a commission. They must be registered with the SEC, pass qualifying exams, and be employed by a broker-dealer firm. A stockbroker charges a commission on each transaction made on the consumer's behalf. Note: Stockbrokers do not have a fiduciary duty to act in your elder's best interest.

There's an App for That!

Research stocks: There are many apps that make researching stocks easier, particularly from mobile devices. Go to your app store and search **Motif. com**, **StockTwits.com**, or **CNN Money**. For more ideas on apps, search for "stock investment."

Track your personal portfolio: To track your personal stock portfolio, ask your broker (e.g., eTrade has an app). Most have apps. Some have advanced features that allow you to scan a product or service barcode and acquire information about the company behind the product, if the company is publicly traded.

CHOOSING THE RIGHT INVESTMENT ADVISOR

Have a Financial Advisor? Great!

There are many investment advisors who can provide objective advice on how to hold investments, asset allocation, retirement income planning, and a host of other financial needs. If your elder already has a trusted financial advisor, great! Have your elder set up a meeting to understand where he is financially. The advisor can tell or remind your elder why financial decisions were made and whether or not any changes are needed. Your elder also can inform the advisor of any health changes and review the decisions made in the past to see if changes should be made going forward.

Need One?

If your elder does not have an investment advisor and feels one is needed, help him carefully select someone who is trustworthy, has your elder's best interest at heart, and is transparent with how he charges for his services.

- Start by asking friends and family for referrals. Get recommendations from people whose financial needs, outlook, or stage of life is similar to that of your elder.
- Research advisors using some online tools. LinkedIn will give you a sense of what each firm is like. See if a particular advisor targets your elder's demographic. The Financial Planning Association also offers a search tool at http://www.plannersearch.org, as does the National Association of Personal Financial Advisors at http://findanadvisor.napfa.org/Home.aspx. Also, check out each recommended firm's company website.

Here are some questions to ask either over the phone or in person during the initial free consultation:

- How do you charge for your services, and how much?
- What licenses, credentials, or other certifications do you have?
- What services do you provide?
- What is the investment approach of the firm? Active or passive investment management?
- Do you accept referral fees?
- Do you have clients similar to me?
- How much contact will I have with you directly?
- Who else will I have contact with in your office?

Note: If one partner managed the couple's investments throughout their life together, your elder may not want to have an advisor step in. Explain to that partner that the other may not have the knowledge he or she has to manage their investments and that it would make sense to get professional help in the event that something happened to the one with the knowledge or experience.

Had a Bad Experience with an Advisor?

Most financial advisors are registered by the state in which they operate or nationally with the SEC. To file a complaint, contact your state's licensing office. You also can contact the North American Securities Administrators Association to find your state's registration office at http://www.nasaa.org. In addition, visit the SEC complaint center at http://www.sec.gov/complaint.shtml for tips on filing a complaint and to help with completing the online form.

Ready Reference for Financial Contacts

Aging Life Care Association: http://www.aginglifecare.org
American Association of Daily Money Managers: http://www.AADMM.com
Attorney General for your state: http://www.naag.org
Centers for Medicare & Medicaid Services website: https://www.cms.gov
Credit Bureaus:
    Experian: http://www.experian.com
    Equifax: http://www.equifax.com
    TransUnion: http://www.transunion.com
Credit Report: https://www.annualcreditreport.com
CFP® Information: http://www.letsmakeaplan.org
CPA Information: http://www.aicpa.org
Federal Healthcare Marketplace: https://www.healthcare.gov
Medicare: https://www.medicare.gov
National Association of Personal Financial Advisors: http://www.napfa.org
National Foundation for Credit Counseling: https://www.nfcc.org
Securities and Exchange Commission: https://www.sec.gov
SHIBA: SHIBA is an organization that protects consumers regarding their health insurance and provides oversight of the insurance industry. Examples of state SHIBA programs can be found at http://www.insurance.wa.gov/ and http://www.oregon.gov/dcbs/insurance/shiba/Pages/shiba.aspx.
Social Security Administration: https://www.ssa.gov
Veterans' ADL Help: http://www.VeteranAid.org
Veterans' Benefits: http://www.benefits.va.gov/benefits

Interesting Opportunity for Free Financial Education

Khan Academy and **Bank of America** are collaborating to offer Bank of America customers as well as noncustomers free, self-paced, easy-to-understand resources to develop better money habits. The resources are available at https://www.bettermoneyhabits.com/khan-academy-partnership.html.

LIVING ENVIRONMENT
PILLAR OF AGING WELLBEING

If you want to identify me . . . ask me not where I live,
or what I like to eat, or how I comb my hair,
but ask me what I think I am living for, in detail,
and ask me what I think is keeping me
from living fully for the thing I want to live for.

—Thomas Merton in *My Argument with the Gestapo*

Chapter Three

MARY JO'S FIRESIDE CHAT

Is Your Elder's Living Environment OK for Living on Her Own?

As children and caring caregivers, we tend to think we know what is best for our elder. We get scared that she will fall, get scammed, or worse, so we ask her to move closer to us, downsize, move in with us, or move into an assisted living home. We tend to overlook that this elder has lived seventy, eighty, even ninety years making her own decisions and determining what's best for her. But, your elder may be showing signs of memory impairment and other concerning diminishment. As the caregiver, you may feel an immense responsibility for her safety and security.

The middle of the road point here is to calibrate with your elder and keep her involved and empowered in making living environment choices. The tension between the caregiver's need for safety and security for the elder eventually bumps head-on into the elder wanting to maintain some form of independence and autonomy. Finding the middle ground is what I focus on as an ALCM and as a certified aging-in-place specialist. I put the elder's desires first and work from there in making all parties comfortable with a care plan regarding the elder's environment. If Mom wants to live independently and has the resources and support to do so, I then build and recommend a care plan that includes appropriate technology, social services, and family support that meets her needs and wants. An elder will usually move to the middle ground and accept help if she knows the alternative is having to sell her home.

A dear friend of mine, Carmela, just turned ninety years old. Her three sons asked me for advice on her living situation. They already have moved her from her home country of Peru to live near two of her three sons. She has a one-floor apartment at street level within a vibrant Spanish community that gathers weekly for social events and games. She also walks several mornings a week with a friend, goes to church every Sunday, and is very involved in the lives of her sons and their families. They see to her every need.

This is quite an idyllic situation, as Carmela has no serious health issues and takes excellent care of herself by swimming, walking, and eating well. She voluntarily gave up her driver's license last year after a few fender-benders. She now takes public transportation or rides with family and friends. In addition, Carmela continues to travel alone to visit family in South America and Europe. She is the model of elderhood for which we should all strive. She takes responsibility for her aging changes, and, as they come, she allows for adaptation and accepts help.

Despite this smart, enthusiastic, vibrant woman's abilities, her sons worry to different degrees about her traveling and living alone. During my assessment of her, she informed me that she wants to live alone until she cannot and that she wants to travel until something changes that prevents her from doing so. In talking with her sons, I shared that there was no reason she should not continue her current level of activities but that perhaps certain safeguards could be built into her travel expeditions. A travel companion, monitoring device, and scheduled check-ins were among some of the ideas I offered. While her current home and living environment allow her to socialize on her terms and to manage her lifestyle, I also suggested that her sons might gain peace of mind if she considered installing security monitoring technology in her home, adding grab bars in the bathroom, and removing throw rugs throughout her home. Carmela has a very realistic view of her future, and she knows life can change in a moment. She is committed to healthy habits and cooperating with her sons as her situation evolves.

Financially, it is best for her to stay in her home for now and bring in services as her needs change. Nonetheless, Carmela and her sons have agreed to revisit the decision on a regular basis. In the meantime, she has a zest for life and for living each moment fully with those she loves.

For the "Living Environment" section of *Eldercare 101*, I have asked Susan Cain McCarty to share the many options for aging in place and alternative living options. Susan is an ALCM, certified senior advisor, and gerontologist who has journeyed with others. She also has made her own living environment transitions. Within this section, she covers the latest information on elder living environments, highlights the importance of putting in place in-home support systems, and details how to have a home assessed for aging-in-place features. Her valuable checklists will help you navigate the choices and what should be considered before changing your elder's living environment.

Living Environment Options
Susan Cain McCarty, MAIS, CSA

Some people speak of aging into older years as a quieter time when most life choices have been made and you can sit back and relax. More often than not, however, the opposite is true. Life beyond age sixty-five can be a busy and sometimes confusing time, particularly if you haven't developed a plan.

Do your parents or other elders for whom you are caring have a plan? Maybe they want to stay in their home but need more support. Perhaps they are considering moving because maintaining the house and yard has become too difficult for them. Maybe their need to move is financially or medically driven. Perhaps they want to live closer to the center of town or join a community of older adults.

Whatever the situation, at some point most elders find themselves at a crossroads requiring changes to their living environment. If they decide to age at home, they may need to hire contractors to make their home safer or homecare aides to help cook, clean, or run errands. If they think an elder community or an assisted living facility is best, how do they find the right place? Investigating options and putting a plan in place is smart!

In this section of *Eldercare 101*, we offer a thoughtful discussion of living environment options, definitions of some confusing terminology, and links to important resources to help you help your aging loved one develop a plan. We truly hope everything we include will assist your elder in navigating her new world as she grows older.

Read on, take notes, and help your elder to consider the ideas we explore. Hopefully, the information will empower your loved one to begin to design a unique plan for living out a full, satisfying life.

AGING AT HOME

Possibly the most significant decision anyone makes in her older years is about where to live. Initially, Mom and Dad may want to ditch the big house and move into a condo on a golf course in Miami. Then, as they age further, they may be less active and possibly suffering losses that require transportation services or help at home. Perhaps they will need more custodial assistance or desire increased interaction with others their age and decide to move to some type of assisted care facility. Elders have many living options today, and their decisions will likely be guided by a combination of values, personal goals, finances, and health.

Despite the multitude of options, 90 percent of surveyed Americans say they want to "age at home." Aging at home is also called "aging in place" and refers to living independently within a community rather than in an assisted living facility. For some, they may age in a home they've lived in for many years—with or without in-home supportive custodial or medical services. For others, aging at home may mean moving to a different home or apartment. This can include living in a home with a group of friends or with adult children. It also can mean living in a "fifty-five and older" community or in a mixed-age community.

In this section, we offer tools to help you help your aging loved ones explore the option of aging at home, with its pros and cons. We also provide links to websites and articles that will assist your elders in finding the support they need for the maintenance of their home as well as their own personal wellbeing.

THE CHOICE

DOES YOUR ELDER WANT TO STAY AT HOME?

It's no surprise that, according to AARP polls, nine out of ten elders say they want to age at home. To live at home, your elder needs to:

- Be able to afford her home and keep it in good repair.
- Know for certain her home is safe.
- Understand and get the help she needs as she ages.

If your elder wants to age at home, there are many questions to ask to determine if doing so is the best option. Having your loved one thoughtfully consider the following and then discuss her answers with you can help her make a good choice.

- Is her home safe and set up to avoid hazards that might cause a fall, a fire, or other potential problems?
- Can she provide the necessary maintenance for her home and yard?
- Can she afford to stay in her home (pay the bills, insurance, home and yard repairs)?
- Is she able to grocery shop and prepare nutritious meals safely?
- Can she perform basic daily tasks including dressing, bathing, cleaning, and cooking?
- If she owns a pet, can she continue to feed, pick up after it, and exercise it?

- Will she have sufficient social interaction if she stays at home? In other words, does she have friends or family who will check on her regularly, if needed, without having the extra effort interfere with her relationships with them?
- Does your elder still drive or have access to transportation?
- Is your elder aware of how to prevent scams from people who come to her home or call her?
- If your elder needs help, is she willing to let volunteers or paid professionals come into her home? If so, how many days per week could she use help?
- If your elder needs custodial or medical support, can she afford qualified in-home caregivers?
- If your elder's memory deteriorates, can she afford twenty-four/seven care?

After going through those questions, ask your elder if staying at home seems like the right or wrong alternative. If, for example, your loved one had more "no" answers than "yes" answers, she might want to explore a retirement community or group home options. Likewise, if she has extensive medical challenges that require doctors, nurses, or therapists on a regular basis, she may need to consider a skilled nursing facility (SNF).

Explore Further

Check out the sections of *Eldercare 101* titled "Getting Help at Home," "Maintaining Your Home," "Life Reimagined," "Transportation Issues," "Emergency Preparedness," "Protection from Scams," and more.

EVER THOUGHT ABOUT
SHARED HOUSING WITH FRIENDS?

While we often shared housing during college or at other times during our younger years, the idea of sharing housing with roommates during our older years rarely occurs to elders. For some older adults, however, this is a good option that can mitigate both social and financial issues. You might want to discuss this possibility with your elders.

If your elders do consider shared housing, they have a variety of options to explore. Would they prefer to move to a new home with other elders who are healthy, living independently, and do not require support? Would they like to invite others into their home to live with them? Would they consider setting up a home for others who require domestic and medical support (in effect, creating their own "adult foster care")? How many roommates and how big of a house would be appropriate to create the environment they envision and that would make financial sense?

Thinking outside the box pays off when exploring the option of shared housing, but there are two definitive considerations: (1) Finding roommates who are a good personality match and, (2) Establishing a legal agreement that provides protection for all parties and addresses worst-case scenarios: What if your Mom doesn't like one of her roommates? What if someone doesn't make timely payments? What if one person doesn't fully contribute to the workload required to maintain the house? And, most importantly, how will your elder get out of the agreement if it doesn't work for her for any reason? Contacting an elder attorney for advice about shared housing contracts would be prudent.

If your elders are considering shared housing, have them answer these questions and discuss their responses with you:

- Do you enjoy interdependence and interaction with others?
- Do you prefer privacy over social interaction?
- Could you envision a shared home that would provide enough privacy?
- Are your current home or apartment expenses too high and burdensome? Could they be significantly reduced through shared housing?
- Are you willing to be transparent and honest about your needs and concerns when entering into a legal agreement?
- Are you willing to downsize your current home and belongings?
- Once you enter into a formal agreement to share housing, can you openly communicate with roommates about any concerns?
- Are you willing to move to another area (city or state) to find the right house or roommate?
- Do you have in mind a particular friend or friends to be your roommates?
- Is the house being considered near shopping, healthcare services, and easy, affordable transportation?

After going through those questions, ask your elder if sharing housing with friends seems like the right or wrong alternative. Explore the pros and cons.

Other Resources

An excellent resource providing information, guidelines, and a sample contract for shared housing is *My House, Our House: Living Far Better for Far Less in a Cooperative Household* by Karen M. Bush, Louise S. Machinist, and Jean McQuillin.

AARP on "House Sharing for Women": http://www.aarp.org/home-fam ily/your-home/info-05-2013/older-women-roommates-house-sharing.html

Baby Boomer Lifeboat: http://www.babyboomerlifeboat.com/baby_boom
er_low_cost_housing.htm

Video about Shared Housing for Elders: https://www.youtube.com/watch
?v=GbXMajUxfsk&feature=youtu.be

IS AN AGE-RESTRICTED COMMUNITY PERFECT?

Age-restricted elder communities have been around a long time. Elders considering senior neighborhoods or communities generally prefer to avoid mixed-age neighborhoods.

Created for people fifty-five and older (age limit varies), these communities may offer both homes and condos. Some communities require that only one person be fifty-five, whereas others require that both be fifty-five or older. The homeowner dues can average $200 to $600 per month and may cover outside home and yard improvements and maintenance as well as upkeep of community properties such as a pool, clubhouse, and golf course. Some charge additional "greens fees" for members who want to golf. In some communities, homeowner dues also pay for road maintenance; the dues, therefore, may be expensive.

On the plus side, many members report feeling safer in an age-restricted community than in a mixed-age neighborhood because the communities are often "gated" and may even have an attendant at the entrance or an automatic gate that requires a security code. Also, there is little traffic and few strangers roaming within the community.

A few concerns should be considered, however, before making this move:

- Most of these communities limit the number of days children may visit. They also may limit the hours the children may be at the pool or in other common areas. This may be of concern for grandparents who enjoy having their grandchildren visit during vacation time.
- Many age-restricted community members complain that the homeowner associations are autocratic and that little oversight exists for setting and enforcing rules, guidelines, and dues.
- Another common complaint is that dues often increase significantly year by year.
- Others complain that "levies" for projects such as road repair are random, though mandatory, and may result in a high, unexpected expense.
- Resale is limited to a small market of adults over fifty-five who prefer age-restricted neighborhoods, so selling may take longer than a home in a mixed-age neighborhood.

When looking at age-restricted communities, be sure your elder asks to see a copy of the rules and guidelines and that she is comfortable with the governing practices and fees. Also, alert your elder to *take a close look at the financial reports of the management company*, or, if this is not made available, be sure she speaks with other homeowners within the community about the viability of the management group. Have your elder ask herself the following questions as well, and have her discuss her responses with you.

- Will you enjoy an older adult community or do you prefer a mixed community with families?
- Are the dues affordable? How much have they varied over the past five years?
- Do you have any say as a homeowner in setting the rules, guidelines, and dues? How much?
- If you can no longer drive, does the community provide public or private access to transportation? If yes, what will that transportation cost?
- Can you "personalize" your outdoor space (garden or yard)? If so, are there any restrictions?
- Is the community near your doctors, hairdresser/barber, friends, faith community, and stores you frequent?

Interested in knowing more? For a list of age-restricted communities, check out http://www.activeadultliving.com/.

WHY NOT MOVE IN WITH YOUR SON OR DAUGHTER?

In many countries, the model of multigenerational families living together is common and expected, and it's not only when the older parents are aging. In the United States, we have gone through phases of multigenerational living—phases that, for the most part, have been economically driven. For example, the 2008 recession triggered an increase in extended families living together. Because living together may be easier if you have independent living quarters, some adult children create alternative living environments such as a "mother-in-law" cottage in the back of the house, a "granny flat" on the basement level, or just a separate entrance. Other adult children even move to a new home more conducive to having a parent live with them or remodel their home, adding on a room or rooms. Although this trend is reversing with the improved economy, in general, as we age, our personal choices, finances, and physical health may guide us toward a decision to live with our children, if that option is available.

One of the pluses of moving in with adult children is that doing so can foster a strong parent-child relationship—but this usually happens only if the parent-child relationship was good throughout life and if everyone is patient throughout an adjustment period. On the other hand, if the parent-child relationship was tumultuous, it's unlikely to change quickly and perhaps will worsen. Setting boundaries when living together also can present a major challenge for both elders and their children; humans are creatures of habit, and moving in together requires that everyone change their habits. Perhaps the toughest hurdle, though, is giving up independence. As reported in AgingCare.com quoting a Gallup and Robinson research report on aging and quality of life, 31 percent of elders said they wouldn't want to live with their children if they could no longer live on their own, whereas 51 percent of the adult children polled said they would be willing to have their parents live with them.[1]

Help your elders to consider the following pros and cons if they are exploring moving in with you or one of your siblings. Also, be sure to agree to "no harm done" if the arrangement doesn't work out for some reason. In fact, this scenario should be discussed in advance and a plan created for options. For example, the elder should know whom she can ask for help outside the family if she needs to call it quits.

Pros of Moving in with Adult Children

- All parties may grow closer through daily interaction.
- Stress may be reduced for everyone—for the adult children, because they feel confident in how they are caring for their parent, and they may not have to drive to check on her. The parent may feel safer, loved, and that her care needs are met.
- Living together can provide an opportunity for the younger generation to learn from their elders and appreciate being in an intergenerational family.
- The elder can create and share family life stories and ensure legacy is passed on to her children (and grandchildren).
- Sharing end-of-life experiences among loved ones can be a beautiful gift to all.
- If the parent can help defray living costs, the adult child may benefit financially with reduced overall expenses.
- If the parent is able, she can help with daily tasks such as light housekeeping, food preparation, and even child care.
- If the elder requires assistance with her ADLs, the adult children may be eligible to receive payment for caregiving services and supplement their income.
- If the parent has home healthcare or custodial care workers coming into the home, the adult children will be able to oversee the care firsthand.

- If the elder is eligible for hospice care and chooses to die at home, the adult children can vigil with their parent in the comfort of their own home where they know their parent is being well loved and cared for until the very end.

Cons of Moving in with Adult Children

- Both elders and their children may feel discouraged if living together isn't immediately easy. For some, the process of adjustment may be a few weeks or months, whereas for others it can be six months or longer.
- If the elder needs a great deal of support on a daily basis, the children may become exhausted.
- Creating private spaces and times in the home may be difficult.
- Costs of retrofitting or renovating the adult child's home to accommodate the parent might be prohibitive.
- Siblings of the son or daughter the parent lives with might feel left out or not believe the elder is receiving the best care or that the elder's money or estate is being mismanaged.
- If the adult children work and the elder needs custodial or healthcare help, having a stranger in the house may cause resentment. Also, the costs for the paid help might be prohibitive.
- If the elder needs help dressing, bathing, or going to the bathroom, she may not be comfortable with her children helping. (If the resources are available, bring in help!)
- Giving up a home and most of your belongings is a difficult adjustment, and the elder may need some grieving time the adult children don't understand because they feel they are giving the elder a gift.
- After seventy, eighty, or ninety years living independently, it's going to be challenging to live with anyone else; this new living situation can leave elders feeling diminished and even without purpose. (This can be true for any move!)
- The elder may have had friends and a sense of community where she previously lived. Now she might feel somewhat isolated and discouraged, as she struggles to find her way around the new community and make new friends.
- In many of today's homes, bedrooms are on the second level; the elder may not be able to negotiate the stairs, so a bedroom might need to be carved out of the living area downstairs, and this can be difficult for everyone.
- Adult children or aging parents may see living together as an opportunity to fix what didn't work well in earlier years, yet this rarely works without counseling.

- Some children are abusive, and some older adults are also abusive toward their children. Be prepared with a plan to ask for help. Talk with a pastor, minister, rabbi, or the local state ombudsman. Be prepared with options if the situation does not work out.
- Some children have been known to take financial advantage of a parent living with them. This is also abuse, and the suggestions in the previous item apply.

Dig Deeper

AARP on "When Parents Move in with Kids": http://www.aarp.org/money/budgeting-saving/info-09-2012/when-parents-move-in-with-kids.html

AARP on "The Financial Implications of Aging Parents Moving In": http://www.aarp.org/home-family/caregiving/info-06-2012/afford-aging-parents-moving-in.html

Agingcare.com article on "How to Handle an Aging Parent's Bad Behavior": http://www.agingcare.com/Articles/bad-behavior-by-elderly-parents-138673.htm

Locating Your Local Ombudsman: http://theconsumervoice.org/get_help

HOW ABOUT JOINING (OR STARTING) A VIRTUAL RETIREMENT COMMUNITY?

Some people are reinventing retirement and creating "virtual retirement communities" (VRCs). This fast-growing option supports independence and, for some, provides more affordable living. The way a VRC works is that your elder stays in her home but she "connects" and contracts with other homeowners to form a "virtual" community.

The first VRC started in Boston in 2001. Some residents decided they wanted the services of a traditional retirement home but also wanted to stay in the house or apartment where they had lived for years. The virtual village they created offered residents handyman assistance whenever they needed it; a ride-sharing system for trips to the dentist, doctor, or dog groomer; and a social network for enjoying the cultural riches that Boston had to offer. Today, more than one hundred VRCs can be found throughout the United States. The NEST (North East Seattle Together) VRC, for example, encompasses fourteen neighborhoods in northeast Seattle. Check it out online at http://www.nestseattle.org.

There are many models of the VRC. What most have in common is a membership or formal contract. When you belong to the VRC, as a member you can be entitled to a variety of cooperative benefits such as transportation, in-home health care, or contractors to repair homes. Membership services may be provided by other members, volunteers within the community, or be paid through VRC dues or by individual members themselves.

Where VRCs differ is the physical model of the "community." In some VRCs, members may live near each other but in a mixed-age community, yet they share services and a common supportive environment. On the other hand, some VRC members live in neighborhoods specifically built for elders within the VRC. Regardless, VRCs are a very clever way to have your cake and eat it, too!

Some questions to have your elder explore if she decides to age at home as part of a VRC:

- Would you enjoy the benefits of having access to qualified contractors and a group of like-minded people as part of your community?
- Would you prefer to stay in your home in a mixed community and be part of a VRC, or would you prefer to be part of a VRC where older adults live in a common neighborhood populated exclusively by elders?
- Are you able to drive, and, if not, does your VRC offer any type of transportation?
- Are the VRC dues affordable, and how much have the fees varied over the past five years?
- Do you see this as a long-term solution or do you think you would need to move again? Is that OK?
- If there isn't a VRC community nearby, would you enjoy starting a new one?

Curious?

Village to Village Network: The "how-tos" of setting up a virtual community; http://www.vtvnetwork.org/

Forbes: Article on virtual retirement communities; http://www.forbes.com/sites/robertlenzner/2013/05/23/socially-minded-seniors-keep-co-op-spirit-alive-in-cambridge/

Fox Business News: Story on the rise of virtual retirement villages; http://www.foxbusiness.com/personal-finance/2013/07/19/rise-virtual-retirement-villages/

Liberty Mutual "The Responsibility Project": Article on a creative solution to retirement homes; http://responsibility-project.libertymutual.com/articles/a-creative-solution-to-retirement-homes

OUTSIDE-THE-BOX HOUSING ALTERNATIVES

Naturally Occurring Retirement Communities

Naturally Occurring Retirement Communities (NORCs) come in every size and makeup as people come up with more and more creative ways for living and aging together. Shared housing and village-type communities are two of the more popular concepts. These ideas place the elder living in multigenerational environments with everyone pitching in to help support the community's needs. Elders play a vital role in supporting the younger generations in these models, which have the added benefits of purposeful living.

NORC organization website: https://www.norcs.org/
Government description of NORC and supportive services: http://aspe. hhs.gov/daltcp/reports/norcssp.htm
U.S. News & World Report **article on NORCS:** http://money.usnews.com/ money/blogs/the-best-life/2009/03/25/is-a-naturally-occurring-retirement-community-right-for-you
Village to Village Network: http://www.vtvnetwork.org/

Tiny Houses and the MEDCottage

A movement taking place across the United States is living in a small footprint to have less impact on the environment or for frugal, simplified living. One adaption is the MEDCottage, http://www.medcottage.com, "a prefabricated 12-by-24-foot bedroom-bathroom-kitchenette unit that can be set up as a free-standing structure in a backyard. It's more than a miniature house. It's decked out with high-tech monitoring and safety features that rival those of many nursing homes." A quick Internet search will yield other emerging ideas for "Tiny Living" for elders.

Tiny House blog: http://tinyhouseblog.com/tiny-house-concept/wonder-cottage-or-granny-pod/
Chicago Tribune **article on MedCottages:** http://www.chicagotribune. com/brandpublishing/primetime/chi-primetime-medcottage-1109 11-story.html
NY Daily News **article on Granny Pods:** http://www.nydailynews.com/ life-style/health/granny-pods-debut-nursing-home-alternative-article-1.12 08916

More Resources on Aging at Home

AARP: Questionnaire with lots of additional video and article links about determining the livability of your home; http://www.aarp.org/livable-communities/info-2014/is-your-home-livable.html

Aging-in-Place (AIP): Website dedicated to those who are aging at home and those who may be helping them; http://aginginplace.com/. For specific tips for aging in place, go to http://aginginplace.com/mini-2/behavioral-adaptations/. For home modification ideas ("universal design"), check out http://aginginplace.com/home-modification/universal-design/.

Certified Aging-in-Place Specialist (CAPS): A certified aging-in-place specialist (CAPS) has been trained through the National Association of Home Builders (NAHB) in the unique needs of the older adult population, aging-in-place home modifications, common remodeling projects, and solutions to common barriers. For more on this program, go to the NAHB website: http://www.nahb.org/directory.aspx?directoryID=188.

Center for Technology and Aging: An organization dedicated to improving the independence of older adults dealing with chronic healthcare issues by promoting the adoption and diffusion of beneficial technologies. See http://www.techandaging.org/index.html for more information.

LeadingAge Center for Aging Services Technology (CAST): An association of six thousand nonprofit organizations leading the charge to expedite the development, evaluation, and adoption of emerging technologies that can improve the aging experience (http://www.leadingage.org/cast.aspx).

The Longevity Network: AARP and United Healthcare team up on this website, http://www.longevitynetwork.org/, to offer information and tools for healthy aging.

National Public Radio (NPR): Story on communities coming together to help people age at home; http://www.npr.org/templates/story/story.php?storyId=129086737

NPR's "Aging at Home: Helping Seniors Stay Put": A series of stories exploring high- and low-tech ways to make it easier for elders to age at home; http://www.npr.org/series/129085934/aging-at-home-helping-seniors-stay-put

National Institute on Aging (NIA): Web page devoted to issues to consider if aging at home; http://www.nia.nih.gov/health/publication/theres-no-place-home-growing-old

THE IN-HOME HELPERS

TYPES OF IN-HOME HELP

Hopefully, your elders can age at home with as little support as possible, but there may be a time when they require in-home care to help with daily activities, medical support, or companionship. Four types of in-home providers address these needs. Typically, people will start with getting help for a few hours once a week to get used to accepting help from others and to identify if the caregiver is a good "fit." Then, as more help is needed, it is easier to increase the help to two times per week, then three times or more per week, or maybe even twenty-four/seven care. When a health professional declares that a person has six months or less to live, the fourth type of in-home provider can be requested.

1. **Home healthcare providers** offer medical support and can be registered nurses, physician's assistants, or other medical professionals.
2. **Custodial care providers** help with daily activities such as bathing, dressing, shopping, light housekeeping and yard work, food preparation and clean up, organizing (personal belongings, calendar, appointments, etc.), and perhaps even driving to and attending appointments.
3. **Companions** can visit, play cards, take walks with elders, and may even drive them to appointments.
4. **Home hospice professionals and volunteers** can provide medical, psychological, and spiritual support at home at the end of life. For more on hospice care, see our "Medical" and "Spiritual" sections.

Home healthcare providers and hospice providers require licensing and adherence to government regulations, as their services can be paid through Medicare benefits. Because custodial care providers may not necessarily be licensed, this section provides ideas on how to select custodial care providers in an effort to offer some guidelines and prevent problematic hiring.

Types of In-Home Custodial Helpers

Caregiver: Assists with daily tasks such as dressing, bathing, cooking, shopping, cleaning, and getting to appointments.

Cleaning service: Cleans interior of home; expectations are set for the level of cleaning. For example, does the fee include windows, interior of refrigerator or oven, or changing bed linens? If so, how often?

House manager: Supervises the ongoing maintenance of a home and the necessary supervision of individuals to ensure the routine functioning and upkeep of a home and its appliances.

Personal chef: Designs, shops for, and prepares meals. These individuals vary in training, background, and nutritional education.

Personal shopper: Given a list of specific needs, will purchase clothes or accessories and deliver to the older adult's residence and charge to the older adult.

Pet care provider and/or groomer: May come to the elder's home to care for any pets.

Links, Links, Links!

AARP on hiring a homecare worker: http://www.aarp.org/relationships/ caregiving-resource-center/info-08-2010/pc_home_care_worker.html

AARP on selecting an agency for in-home care: http://www.aarp.org/ relationships/caregiving-resource-center/info-10-2010/pc_choosing_an_ agency_for_inhome_care_video.html

AARP on types of in-home care providers: http://www.aarp.org/relationships/ caregiving-resource-center/info-08-2010/pc_in-home_care_providers.html

Background checks (important if you hire an individual rather than contracting with an agency): http://www.top10bestbackgroundcheck. com/?kw=background%20checking&c=45528255028&t=search&p=&m =p&adpos=1t2&dev=c&devmod=&mobval=0&ts=c&a=467&gclid=CIL k5Z_M88ECFZNhfgodkDoAaw

Companions and activities: Fact sheet to help you explore your options. Also, consider contacting your senior community center or look into adult day care options in your area. http://www.seniorcenterdirectory.com/, or http://www.eldercare.gov/Eldercare.NET/Public/Resources/Factsheets/ Adult_Day_Care.aspx

Comparison of hospitals, doctors, and home healthcare services: Government collected data on hospitals, doctors, services, and other issues. Compare services, interact with the data, and download at https://data. medicare.gov/.

Eldercare locator: 1-800-677-1116 or http://www.eldercare.gov/Eldercare. NET/Public/Index.aspx

Federal government fact sheet about home health care: http://www. eldercare.gov/Eldercare.NET/Public/Resources/Factsheets/Home_Health_ Care.aspx

Home healthcare and hospice locator: http://www.nahcagencylocator.com/
Home services locator and comparison: https://www.medicare.gov/home
  healthcompare/
Paying for home health care: http://longtermcare.gov/costs-how-to-pay/
Questions to ask an in-home care provider: http://www.nahc.org/con
  sumer-information/right-home-care-provider/
Specialists caring for elders with Alzheimer's disease: http://www.alz.org/
  carefinder

There's an App for That!

For the average pricing of in-home care services in your area, check out the
Genworth Cost of Care app at https://www.genworth.com/corporate/about-
genworth/industry-expertise/cost-of-care.html.

For **"My Personal Care Team"** and **"My Home Team"** forms to use for
keeping track of addresses, phone numbers, e-mail addresses, and the like, of
people and organizations that are supporting your elder's aging-at-home decision, go to https://rowman.com/ISBN/9781442265462.

CHECKLIST OF THINGS WITH WHICH I NEED HELP

Go over this list with your elder to help her assess her needs. Although it is
not comprehensive, it will at least get your elder thinking about how an in-
home custodial caregiver can make her life easier.

HEALTH
- Exercise
  - Taking walks
  - Stretching
  - Strength exercises
  - Brain exercises
  - Other

EATING
- Grocery shopping
  - Driving to the grocery store
  - Picking up grocery bags

- o Putting groceries away
- o Other
- Food Preparation
  - o Breakfast
  - o Lunch
  - o Dinner
  - o Preparing meals ahead and freezing
  - o You decide on menu/pick recipes
  - o Have caregiver be main cook
  - o Assist you in the kitchen
  - o Other
- Cleanup
  - o Wash/stack/dry dishes
  - o Put dishes away
  - o Keep refrigerator cleared of "old" food
  - o Keep kitchen cupboards organized
  - o Clean stove/oven/microwave
  - o Clean sink and counter
  - o Put away dish towels/sponges
  - o Other

DAILY LIVING
- Hygiene
  - o Showering/bathing
  - o Dressing
  - o Washing hair
  - o Shaving
  - o Nail care (hands or feet)
  - o Other
- Financial
  - o Pay bills that can't be paid online
  - o Organize receipts/tax pertinent information
  - o Other
- Home Cleaning
  - o Light housekeeping
  - o Laundry
  - o Ironing
  - o Changing bed linens
  - o Organizing recycling
  - o Gathering and taking out the trash
  - o Other

- Organizing
  - Mail
  - Bills
  - Calendar
  - Planning appointments (doctor, hair, nails, etc.)
  - Planning outings (trips, plays, etc.)
  - Other
- Medical
  - Tracking appointments (calendar, give reminders, etc.)
  - Accompanying to appointments (PCP, specialists, etc.)
  - Drive you there or meet you there
  - Gather concerns from you and from your family members to discuss during appointment
  - Take notes and send to pertinent family members
  - Medications (including insulin, oxygen, and eye, ear and on-the-skin medication)
  - Get updated prescription list from PCP
  - Help fill pill dispenser
  - Track if medications are taken/prescriptions are filled
  - Other
  - Treatments prescribed by the PCP (including colostomy, bladder catheters, wound care, etc.)
- Social
  - Play games
  - Eat out
  - Organize dates with friends
  - Other
- Transportation
  - Car maintenance (if still driving)
  - Direction help for appointments/outings
  - Caregiver drive you places (errands, shopping, appointments, worship services, events/classes, etc.)
  - Help orchestrating transportation (especially low-cost for elders)
  - Other
- Pet Care (if appropriate)

SELECTING IN-HOME CUSTODIAL CARE PROVIDERS

Note: See our "Medical" section for more on home *health*care providers and services. This checklist is intended to help you find help with your elder's *nonmedical* or custodial needs.

- Assess your elder's needs. Create a written list of activities with which she needs help (e.g., cooking, cleaning, grocery shopping, driving to doctors' appointments, paying bills). Perhaps the last section helped your elder to get started on this list.
- Consider whether your elder wants to contract directly with a person or whether she wants to hire the in-home care provider through an agency. Inviting an individual into the home rather than going through an agency to hire the provider can put your elder at risk for theft and abuse. Most agencies do thorough background checks, and the agency can be held responsible for abuse, theft, and the like.
- Check with friends and relatives and ask for referrals for individuals as well as agencies.
- Check out various websites such as https://www.care.com. You can find these by searching online "caregiver [plus city and state]." Craigslist.org is also another good place to look for individuals as well as agencies. Find your local Craigslist by searching online for "Craigslist.org [plus your city and state]."
- If choosing an agency, ask if the organization conducts background checks. It's surprising that many states do not have laws requiring agencies to perform a background check on their employees.
- If using an agency, find out if the agency will allow interviews of a few candidates and then request the person who best fits with your elder's personality and will meet her needs. Having a number of choices is best, because your elder needs to feel absolutely comfortable with the caregiver.
- If the agency-provided caregiver is a good fit and this seems like a long-term fit, an option is to "buy out" the contract and employ the caregiver directly. Check out the contract in advance and understand all options.
- When contracting privately with an individual, your elder will be considered an "employer" and will be responsible for provider payroll taxes and insurance, in case of injury. This may be covered under your elder's homeowner's insurance policy, so you will definitely want to check with her insurance provider. Also, check out "HomePay" on https://www.care.com for online support in caregiver payroll management and tax filing.
- When contracting someone as an "employer," talk with an elder attorney in advance to understand any legal ramifications.
- When hiring an individual directly, request a resume and several professional references. You or your elder should check all references! If possible, also run a background check. Check out this link for information on paid services for employer background checks: http://www.top10bestbackgroundcheck.com/?kw=background%20checking&c=45528255028&t=s

earch&p=&m=p&adpos=1t2&dev=c&devmod=&mobval=0&ts=c&a=4
67&gclid=CILk5Z_M88ECFZNhfgodkDoAaw.

- Ask to see the applicant's current business license. Conduct online searches to see if any negative reviews or complaints show up.
- Whether using an agency or hiring directly, determine, based on your elder's needs, if you should consider hiring more than one provider. Some in-home care providers specialize in some types of care and others will provide a variety of care services.
- Based on what they will specifically do for your elder, discuss the hours and cost with the service providers. Is their pay set according to number of hours? If so, what is the hourly rate? Are there a minimum number of hours? Many caregivers charge more for less than twenty hours or if you use them "on call."
- Can you or your elder call them as needed or do the caregivers need to adhere to a specific schedule?
- What happens if a care provider is sick or doesn't show up?
- What happens on weekends, nights, or holidays? Do the fees change? If so, what are the specific costs?
- Are they able and willing to provide transportation? Some won't be insured and can't transport your elder.
- Is your elder willing to let the care providers drive her car to transport her to and from appointments, to go grocery shopping, and so on? If so, check into having the care providers insured on your elder's car.
- If the care providers are willing to transport your elder or run her errands, will they charge an additional fee?
- Will they honor client confidentiality?
- Be comfortable explaining what your elder needs and wants—both to the provider agency and the individuals. For example, if you and your elder don't want the in-home care providers on social media or watching movies during their time with your elder, make that desire clear.
- Using an ALCM can make this process easier!

For a form to use for keeping track of addresses, phone numbers, e-mail addresses, and the like, of **"Potential In-Home Helpers,"** go to https://rowman.com/ISBN/9781442265462.

Hiring Caregivers through an Agency vs. Hiring Privately

Here are a few considerations when you are trying to decide which direction to go. Before making a final decision, be sure to consult your elder law attorney, financial planner, or CPA.

	HOME CARE AGENCY	HIRE PRIVATELY
Locates and hires the caregiver and assesses for competency	Agency does	By family
Does the background screening, reviews business and personal references, screens for illegal drug use	Agency does*	By family. Private individuals can access background checks through local government enforcement agencies.
Provides ongoing training/education	Agency does*	Caregiver responsible
Responsible for caregiver's benefits, etc.	Agency does*	By family
Supervises caregiver's care and the services provided	Agency does	By family
Provides back-up caregivers when someone calls off because of illness, injury, and/or personal emergency	Agency does	Unlikely, unless family has hired more than one caregiver who is able to step in and cover
Tasks caregivers able to perform	Agency regulates (generally, most caregivers are not permitted to drive clients)	Greater flexibility and generally less restriction

	HOME CARE AGENCY	HIRE PRIVATELY
Time it takes for caregiving services to begin	Generally, a licensed nurse is required to assess the client and set up plan of care before caregiver can start.	No restrictions other than family's ability to locate caregivers
"On-call" caregiving	Many agencies provide unscheduled or on-call care if they have caregivers available, but they will generally charge more.	Families would need to scramble to call family members, friends, or other substitute caregivers they personally know, and substitute caregivers would probably charge more than the normal rate.
Cost of care	Varies; rate determined by agency and/or registry	Varies depending upon the caregiver, who sets own rate
Time caregiver can work	Generally, shifts are 4, 6, 8, or 12 hours	Shifts vary depending on what the caregiver is willing to do and negotiates with family.
Ability to negotiate on rates/costs	Agency generally not able to negotiate different rates	Family can negotiate based on need; some families offer room and board or use of car as partial payment for services.
Other paperwork (county, state, and/or federal taxes)	Agency does	Consult with a tax specialist

* Note: Check your particular state's regulations, as home care agency and/or registry rules vary from state to state.

THE MAINTENANCE

THINGS TO CONSIDER IN KEEPING UP WITH THE HOUSE

If your elders are aging at home, their house must not only be safe, but it also must be maintained inside and out. Depending upon the health and ability of your elders, they might manage some repairs and maintenance on their own or enlist the help of family members or friends. Some home chores, such as cleaning the roof, elders should never attempt on their own! But hiring outside contractors and workers can be scary—and accepting that we can't do everything we did when we were younger can be frustrating. It would help if we all started using support services when we are in our fifties to be accustomed to having help in our seventies.

To find home maintenance support for your elders, ask an ALCM. Or check with the National Association of Homebuilders (NAHB) to find a certified aging-in-place specialist (CAPS) to assist your elders in determining necessary repairs and in finding the right people to support them. The NAHB website is a great resource: http://www.nahb.org/directory.aspx?sectionID=1391&directoryID=188.

In the meantime, here's a quick list of things to consider as you assist your elders in keeping up with their home:

Indoor Regular Maintenance

Your elders, a volunteer, a paid housekeeper, or a home care aide will want to take care of daily tasks including:

- Dusting, vacuuming, cleaning sinks and toilets, and filling and emptying the dishwasher (or washing and drying the dishes)
- Laundry
- Changing and laundering bedding
- Taking out the trash
- Pet care including feeding, brushing, walking, and cleaning up the yard or the litter box

Indoor "As Needed" Maintenance

While your elders may be capable of easy maintenance such as changing lightbulbs or fixing a loose drawer pull, they probably will need to hire help or find a volunteer to take care of some indoor maintenance tasks such as:

- Painting and deeper cleaning of windows, blinds, other window coverings, and light fixtures
- Checking for any mold, air, or water leaks
- Repairs to keep windows and doors in safe, working condition
- Plumbing, electrical repairs for heating and air conditioning systems, appliance maintenance, and installing strategic lighting sources
- Having the fireplace (if applicable) inspected, cleaned, and, if necessary, serviced annually

Outside Regular Maintenance

- Keeping gutters clean and in repair
- Keeping sidewalks clear of debris, snow, or ice
- Mowing any lawn areas
- Weeding garden beds
- Raking leaves as needed

Outside "As Needed" Maintenance

- Siding and roof repair
- Landscape care (especially annual or semiannual care and pruning of trees to ensure they are healthy and safe)
- Cleaning and repairing windows and screens
- Painting
- Covering faucets before freezing weather
- Repairing any cracks in steps and concrete
- Building and maintaining stair rails and ramps

Resources on Paying for the Home and Its Upkeep

Consider deferring your property taxes: Contact your elder's county tax agency and ask if it has a deferral program for elders.

Housing and Urban Development (HUD) on getting financial help to pay for home repairs: http://portal.hud.gov/hudportal/HUD?src=/topics/home_improvements, or call the Public and Indian Housing (PIH) Customer Service Center at 1-800-955-2232 for the phone number of your local HUD office.

Housing & Urban Development (HUD) on reverse mortgages: http://www.hud.gov/offices/hsg/sfh/hcc/hcs.cfm.

Habitat for Humanity: They not only build new homes for people who can't afford homes, but some chapters also perform repairs for elders; http://www.habitat.org/local/affiliate?zip=Enter+zip+code&country=US.

National Council on Aging (NCOA) on home equity or reverse mortgages: http://www.ncoa.org/enhance-economic-security/home-equity/, or call 1-855-899-3778 for objective counseling on reverse mortgages and advice for how to stay in your home.

More Resources on Home Repair and Modification

AARP Livable Communities Guides (English and Spanish): Tips on keeping your home safe and in good condition and ideas on low-cost or no-cost home improvements; http://www.aarp.org/livable-communities/publications/

Angie's List: A paid subscription-supported website containing crowd-sourced reviews of local businesses; http://www.angieslist.com.

Federal government on home repair and modification: http://www.elder care.gov/eldercare.net/public/resources/topic/Home_Repair.aspx

Federal Trade Commission on selecting a contractor: http://www.con sumer.ftc.gov/articles/0242-hiring-contractor

National Association of Home Builders (NAHB): Directory to find CAPS as well as remodelers and contractors who specialize in the aging-at-home market; http://www.nahb.org/directory.aspx?sectionID=1391&dire ctoryID=188

TOP TEN TIPS FOR REDUCING HAZARDS AT HOME

Falls are the leading cause of injury among older adults, and, sadly, six out of ten falls happen at home! Falls often can be the incident that forces an elder to leave her home and move to a more supportive environment. That said, many things can be done to create a home that is as free from hazards as possible. Here are some tips about how to create a safe home.

1. Remove all throw and area rugs. This is the most common and inexpensive fix! Carpeting should be low pile with firm pads and a smooth, slip-resistant surface.
2. If using or anticipating using a walker or wheelchair, ideally hallways and doorways should be thirty-two to thirty-six inches wide for easy passage.
3. Install handrails on both sides of *all* stairways.
4. A one-story home is ideal, but for houses with multilevels, consider a motorized stairlift. Check out Acorn http://www.acornstairlifts.com and Bruno http://www.bruno.com/stairlifts-home.html, the best-known manufacturers of stairlifts. Note: Permits are required for even residential installation of stairlifts; usually the installer takes care of the permits, but be sure to ask.

5. The ideal height for a toilet is two and a half inches higher than standard toilets. Look for toilets advertised as "comfort height" toilets.
6. Install a fold-down seat in the shower and have a long, flexible hose on the showerhead.
7. Provide adequate lighting in the bathroom and shower. The new Nest Protect fire alarms have motion night lights built in. Check out their website at https://nest.com/smoke-co-alarm/life-with-nest-protect.
8. Ensure that the tub, shower, and bathroom floors have nonslip surfaces. In fact, pay attention to floor slip ratings for every surface in the home including patios and decks.
9. Install grab bars that will support 250–300 lbs. in the shower, near the bathtub, by the toilet, in hallways, and near handrails.
10. Install handrails along any ramps. Also, ramps shouldn't be too steep. Recommendation: No greater than one-inch rise for each twelve inches in length.

Additional Safety Tips

- Double check that all smoke detectors are in working order.
- Be sure there is at least one CO_2 detector in the home.
- Install working, easy-to-use locks on all windows and doors.

In case of a fall, it's good to have a personal emergency response system (PERS) in place. Check out http://www.mylively.com for small sensor-based, user-installed and managed technology.

HIGH-TECH AGING AT HOME

In-home sensor-based technology will be the key to the future of safely aging at home. Sensors are typically small devices installed on doors, stoves, ovens, refrigerators, under mattresses, and on medication dispensers. The devices record when an elder opens and closes doors and when she turns burners and ovens on and off. They weigh the elder when she lies down. Alerts are sent if the elder leaves the house and doesn't return within a "normal" amount of time or if the refrigerator door is left open. For example, a simple door sensor allows caregivers a better night's sleep when monitoring a loved one with dementia. Some systems "learn" habits of an elder and send an alert if the person changes behaviors. Most of these systems also include a personal device—typically a wristband. Much of the technology comes out of a GE and Intel partnership. One early-entry commercial provider is **Live!y** (http://

www.mylively.com). For other providers, search online for "eldercare sensor based monitoring" or "sensor-based healthcare for elders." Right now, this technology is not broadly available, is technically complex, requires professional installation and monitoring, and is too expensive for many. For the "ideal" home, see "Universal Design" at the NAHB's website at http://www.nahb.org/generic.aspx?genericContentID=89934.

More Resources on Creating a Safe Home

CDC—National Center for Injury Prevention and Control: Article on fall prevention; http://www.cdc.gov/ncipc/pub-res/toolkit/ChecklistforSafety.htm

CDC—National Center for Disease Control and Prevention: Listings of different types of emergencies and tips for preparing and safety; http://www.bt.cdc.gov/disasters/index.asp

Find a certified specialist in "home design" to advise on home safety: http://www.nahb.org/directory.aspx?sectionID=0&directoryID=188

Live!y: Company offering medical alert systems and devices; www.mylively.com

Mayo Clinic: Great web page on fall prevention; http://www.mayoclinic.org/healthy-living/healthy-aging/in-depth/fall-prevention/art-20047358

MedLine Plus: On the importance of exercise and program suggestions; http://www.nlm.nih.gov/medlineplus/exerciseforseniors.html

NAHB: Directory to help you find certified aging-in-place specialists to assess your home for safety and comfort; http://www.nahb.org/directory.aspx?sectionID=1391&directoryID=188

National Safety Council: Web page on fall-proofing your home; http://www.nsc.org/safety_home/HomeandRecreationalSafety/Falls/Pages/OlderAdultFalls.aspx

Nest Protect: Company offering home safety products; https://nest.com

WebMD: Web page on making your home fall proof; http://www.webmd.com/healthy-aging/making-your-home-fall-proof

EATING WELL AT HOME

If your elders are aging at home, they may find they don't have the energy to spend lots of time shopping for and preparing meals. Thus, they may end up eating less nutritious meals than they should. Adequate food and nutritious food are at the center of an elder's ability to continue to successfully age at home!

Many community organizations offer food programs. Government programs are also available for those who qualify for aid. One such program is the Supplemental Nutrition Assistance Program (SNAP), formerly the Food Stamp Program.

Today, many people have care providers shop for groceries as part of their duties. Some elders receive assistance from friends and fellow parishioners. If your elder has such support, ask these people to provide meals that can be frozen and stored—in addition to eaten fresh.

Also, many grocery stores will deliver, and some have online ordering. For information about ordering groceries online and setting up delivery, search online for "free grocery delivery" or the name of your elder's local grocer, or call your elder's local grocer for more information.

Check Out These Resources

Eldercare.gov: General information about nutrition and dietary guidelines for the elderly; http://www.eldercare.gov/eldercare.net/public/resources/topic/Food_Nutrition.aspx#national

Meals on Wheels Association of America: http://www.mowaa.org/

Older Americans Act (OAA) Nutrition Program: http://www.aoa.acl.gov/AoA_Programs/HCLTC/Nutrition_Services/index.aspx

Senior Centers: Many offer meals on specific days; http://www.seniorcenter-directory.com and https://www.ncoa.org/national-institute-of-senior-centers/

SNAP: http://www.nutrition.gov/food-assistance-programs/supplemental-nutrition-assistance-program

SNAP's pre-screening eligibility: http://www.snap-step1.usda.gov/fns/

U.S. Dept. of Health and Human Services, Administration for Community Living (AOA): Find government agencies to help with most aging issues; www.aoa.gov/AoA_programs/OAA/How_To_Find/Agencies/find_agencies.aspx

LIVING OPTIONS WITH BUILT-IN SUPPORT

Whereas most people say they want to age at home, some will prefer living in facilities that provide the option for more support. Some will make this choice because they desire more social interaction than is available to them in their home setting. Some say they feel safer living in an assisted-care environment. Or perhaps they need medical help and their LTC insurance benefits will only pay benefits if they live in a facility. Increasingly, LTC insurance will provide support both at home and in a facility, but check your elder's policy.

Also, boredom, loneliness, and depression are often feelings stereotypically associated with elders living in facilities. But these stereotypes do not have to be true—if proper due diligence is made during the selection process.

For example, look for Eden Alternative (http://www.edenalt.org) care facilities or "Green Houses" (http://www.thegreenhouseproject.org). These highly respected facilities focus on relationships and are filled with plants, animals, gardens, and the intimate lifestyle found in a real home.

In this section, we discuss assisted-care types of homes and offer tips and resources for further exploration. Nursing homes, skilled nursing facilities, and rehab facilities are discussed in our "Medical" section. For a ready reference about nursing homes, check out http://www.medicare.gov/nursinghome compare/search.html. We feature this information with the hope that what you and your elders learn will empower your family to make the best choices for the future of your aging loved ones.

There's an App for That!

For the average pricing of assisted care facilities in your elder's area, check out the **Genworth Cost of Care app** at https://www.genworth.com/corporate/about-genworth/industry-expertise/cost-of-care.html.

CONSIDERING A CONTINUUM OF CARE

As our elders age, many likely will need some form of support—whether it is custodial or medical. If that support is available in the home as we discussed in the last section, great. If not, various other living environment options are available that can be categorized as two types of businesses:

1. One is based on *living enhancements* and are referred to as "assisted-living" types of homes:
   o Adult foster care homes
   o Continuing care retirement communities
   o Assisted living facilities
   o Memory care facilities
2. The other is based on *medical needs*:
   o Nursing homes
   o Skilled nursing facilities
   o Inpatient rehabilitation facilities
   o Hospice facilities

But lines of these facilities blur. For example, in continuing care retirement communities and some assisted living facilities, elders can stay where they are from independent living all the way through needing skilled nursing care or memory care. Also, there may be skilled nursing care offered at memory care facilities.

Given the distinction, though, of *living enhancement* versus *medical needs*, it is critical that your elder know the rules and regulations governing the facility she chooses. Despite all the warmth and caring the facility staff might convey to prospective residents, facilities are businesses and can't remain in business unless they are profitable. With this in mind, be sure your elder understands under what conditions she could be moved from one section of a facility to another and under what conditions she could be required to leave. For example, if your elder runs out of money, will she have to leave the facility or does the facility have "Medicaid beds"—beds certified eligible for Medicaid payment? Or will you, siblings, or someone else need to foot the bill? And, can you afford it? Also, what happens if your elder is living at an adult foster home and becomes medically fragile or needs memory care? Does she have a Plan B for a nursing home or a memory care facility?

Because where your elder lives out her elder years is such an important but confusing decision, we highly recommend seeking the help of an ALCM to sort through the options. To get started on the decision process, though, we share in this section the main characteristics of each of the "assisted-living" options.

As noted earlier, the medical facilities will be discussed in our "Medical" section.

For More Information

AARP's Long-term Care Calculator: http://www.aarp.org/relationships/ caregiving-resource-center/LTCC.html

Federal State and County Resources: This highly recommended web page can help you locate many state and county resources on aging. 1-800-677-1116, http://www.eldercare.gov/Eldercare.NET/Public/Index.aspx

OVERVIEW OF ASSISTED-LIVING TYPES OF HOMES

Typically, there are four main options when someone is exploring living in an assisted-care environment:

1. **Adult foster care homes** (private homes typically providing rooms for two to ten elders)
2. **Assisted living facilities** (ALFs)
3. **Continuing care retirement communities** (CCRCs)
4. **Memory care facilities** (Although some memory care facilities are stand-alone facilities, they are also often included within ALFs and CCRCs.)

Factors Involved in Choosing

Within these options are a range of variations including level of support, size of facility, whether the place accepts Medicare or Medicaid, and, of course, the important "location, location." Do your elders want to live in a neighborhood near you, your siblings, their doctors, or their faith community? Should they be in the heart of town with easy access to transportation?

Another factor in choosing where to live involves the potential for **extent of care needed**. For example, consider the following:

- Perhaps your elder requires insulin or another type of subcutaneous injection (shot given into the fat layer between the skin and muscle). Does the facility have staff qualified to administer such an injection on a regular basis?
- What if your elder needs a two-person transfer or the use of a Hoyer Lift (mechanical lift). Is the facility equipped for this?
- Does the facility offer night care?

Continuum of care is another factor to consider. That is, should your elders look for an assisted-living situation where they start out living independently but can gradually take advantage of more and more custodial or medical support? What happens if one of your loved ones eventually suffers from dementia or Alzheimer's disease? Does the assisted living facility she has selected have a memory unit, or will your loved one have to make another move to a dedicated memory care facility? What about hospice care at the end of life? Is that available?

Very specific considerations might also need to be taken into account when choosing the right place for your elder to live. Depending upon your particular elder, in your search do you need to address:

- Language of origin
- America Sign Language ability of staff
- Braille availability
- Racial or cultural considerations
- LGBT considerations

Restriction Considerations

To move into a care facility, your elder will participate in "an intake process" that often includes an assessment of her ADLs, medications, medical requirements, and other demographic information. Requirements and restrictions vary from facility to facility. Some possible restrictions include but aren't limited to:

- Smoking
- Drug use—illegal or prescription drug abuse
- Use of medical marijuana
- Alcohol use or abuse
- Pets
- Behaviors that are uncontrollable such as aggression; strong, vulgar language; exit seeking; and wandering (into other resident's rooms)

When it comes to making the decision about where your elder should live, the choices, options, and considerations are numerous—and can be overwhelming. Once again, we recommend contacting an ALCM to help sort out the possibilities and to find the right fit.

Valuable Resource

Where Should I Live When I Retire? by Bernice Hunt. Available on Amazon. com and at other bookstores.

ADULT FOSTER CARE HOMES (ADULT CARE HOMES)

Although not all states have adult foster care homes, those that do determine what, if any, license and training is required. Oregon, for example, is a pioneer in alternative care models and offers three levels of licensing for adult foster care homes. These levels dictate a specific type of experience required for those owning the adult foster home and working there. In general, however, most adult foster care homes:

- Are single-family residences with the owners or hired care providers living in the home with the residents.
- Offer a "homelike" environment.
- House between two and ten elders (maximum number is determined by each state).
- Are considerably less expensive than assisted living facilities but have fewer amenities.
- Provide supervised custodial care, meals, and laundry services.
- Expect the elder to be ambulatory and to be able to perform personal hygiene with minimal supervision. A few but not many adult care homes accept people who need significant care.
- Permit wheelchairs. Some adult care homes do not permit wheelchairs.
- Are possibly licensed to dispense medications.
- Provide minimal, if any, medical support.
- Provide transportation to medical appointments and outside activities. Some adult care homes do not provide transportation.

Due Diligence

Check with your state Area Agency on Aging (AAA) or Department of Human Services (DHS) to find out if your state has adult foster care homes. If they do, ask if they license and inspect the adult foster homes, how often they inspect, whether they can provide information on complaints, and how these complaints are resolved. To find your local AAA or DHS, go to: http://www.eldercare.gov/Eldercare.NET/Public/Index.aspx or http://www.aoa.gov/AoA_programs/OAA/How_To_Find/Agencies/find_agen cies.aspx?sc=OR.

Get Another Opinion from an ALCM

Given the importance of this housing and care provider decision and the lack of a "standard" for what will be provided from an adult foster care provider, hiring an ALCM to thoroughly research your elder's adult foster care home options may be a good decision. ALCMs are professionals and impartial when offering recommendations. They do not receive compensation from the homes they recommend. To find an ALCM, go to http://www. aginglifecare.org.

Even More Info

AARP fact sheet on adult foster care: http://www.aarp.org/home-garden/ housing/info-03-2010/fs174.html
For more information on adult foster care homes in your area, search online for "adult foster care [plus state]."

DOES ADULT FOSTER CARE FEEL RIGHT?

Adult foster care homes offer many models—from nearly independent living where the home is more of a "group home" and the residents have a high degree of autonomy, to a model where the residents require assistance with daily tasks of living. Some are run by nurses and can offer medical support. Some even care for residents requiring memory care.

Whereas adult foster care homes can't offer many of the amenities that large assisted care facilities can, many elders choose them because they are small, quiet, more personalized environments and because they are considerably less expensive than large assisted care facilities. In addition, some adult foster care owners specialize in a type of care or a type of elder who would live with them: for example, men only, women only, memory care, ambulatory. This makes the option attractive if your elder has specific needs or preferences.

If your elder is thinking of moving to an adult foster care home, explore these questions with her to help to determine if adult foster care is the right choice—at least for the time being.

- Would you prefer living in a smaller place such as an adult care home with only a few older adults rather than living in a larger facility with many residents, staff, and activities?
- Would you enjoy and participate in arranged outings and the activities offered by the homeowners?
- Will the adult care home owners or managers provide transportation to appointments and outings? If not, can friends and family members provide transportation?
- Do you want to be in a "home environment," where you live in close proximity to others, as though you are part of the same family?
- Will you be OK to eat whatever is being made for food on any given day?
- Will you be required to share a room or will you have your own room?
- Will you feel as though you have enough privacy?
- Will you feel safe?
- Will family members and friends feel welcome any time?
- Do you have enough money to pay the fees to stay at the adult foster home? If so, how long will the money last or will Medicaid be a consideration?
- Will you be comfortable moving again to another facility if you need more support than the adult foster care home can afford?
- Do you have any special needs (medical, mental, or physical) that will narrow down the adult care home choices you have? If so, what are they?

Once your elder has answered these questions and discussed her answers with you, explore finishing this phrase: "Adult foster care seems right or wrong because _____ ."

CHOOSING AN ADULT FOSTER CARE HOME

If your elder is considering adult foster care, get referrals from aging friends, family members, and the staff at a local senior center. Also, ask social workers at nursing homes and hospitals for recommendations as well as check with your county Area Agency on Aging to find out if particular homes are licensed and if complaints have been filed against them. Then visit the top suggestions with your elder and compare several homes. Here are some suggested questions and topics your elder can consider during visits:

- Is the provider friendly and open? Does she listen carefully to you?
- Do you think she will be open to your comments and encourage your maximum independence?

- Does she introduce you to the current residents? Is the provider respectful to you and the residents?
- Are the residents friendly and people with whom you would enjoy spending time?
- Who is the "staff," and who is at the home during the day and at night? Who comes when the typical staff are on vacation, ill, or unable to work for personal reasons? Remember, you are living in a small environment, so you will want to feel comfortable both with the owner, other residents, and any staff.
- Is the home clean, neat, and organized?
- Does the home smell pleasant?
- Does the home have activity areas or centers such as a TV area with DVDs; a place to play cards or read outside your room; a patio or deck; a nice yard; or a safe neighborhood for taking walks?
- Can you walk to stores and parks or other desired destinations?
- Is transportation provided to appointments, to your place of worship, and for other personal errands?
- Is the home in close proximity to your friends and relatives?
- Can your friends and family visit unannounced and during reasonable hours?
- Can your friends and family take you off-site in their vehicles? For some adult care homes, this can be an insurance risk.
- Are you LGBT? If so, let the adult care home provider know and ask if she has had other LGBT residents and how they feel about you as an LGBT person.
- Are pets welcomed? This may be a positive or a negative for you.
- What are the monthly fees and what situations would cause the fees to increase (e.g., extended care)?
- Under what conditions might you be asked to leave, and how much notice will be provided?
- Can you remain if you outlive your resources and are dependent on Medicaid?
- If the home isn't licensed to provide medical support, does a nurse come to dispense medication and perform routine blood pressure and heart rate screening?

For a form to use for keeping track of addresses, phone numbers, e-mail addresses, first impressions, and the like, of **"Potential Adult Foster Care Homes,"** go to https://rowman.com/ISBN/9781442265462.

BLURRING OF THE LINES:
CONTINUING CARE RETIREMENT
COMMUNITIES AND ASSISTED LIVING FACILITIES

The terms *continuing care retirement communities* (CCRC) and *adult living facilities* (ALFs) are often used interchangeably, and, indeed, their models are becoming more similar. If you search online for "adult living facility," you will find facilities that are both CCRCs and ALFs (by traditional definition). Therefore, be sure you know what you want and for what you are paying. In the next pages, we provide a textbook definition of CCRC and ALF, but, again, remember that many use these terms interchangeably.

A CCRC used to require a high buy-in of anywhere from $100,000 to $1 million, and many but not all offered four levels of support: independent living, assisted care, medical care, and memory care. Their financial model could be the same fee no matter how long one lived there; or specific service levels; or pay as you go. Today, however, the buy-in is not required in all CCRCs, although many still do require this. For those that don't charge an up-front buy-in, the financial models are similar to many ALFs.

Initially, ALFs did not offer independent living or memory care but did offer assisted care and medical care. Today, many, although not all, ALFs offer all four levels of care. Most ALFs do not require a high buy-in, but always ask for specific information in writing about levels of care and cost models.

CONTINUING CARE RETIREMENT COMMUNITIES

The traditional model of a CCRC is a facility that offers four levels of care: Independent living; nonmedical support or "assisted living"; medical care; and memory care. CCRCs often but not always require a buy-in that can be anywhere from $100,000 to $1 million, together with a monthly fee of anywhere from $3,000 to $7,000. Of those that have a buy-in fee, how these are handled is different from one facility to the next. Sometimes the fee is nonrefundable; other times, some of the fee is returned to the elder's estate upon death. The fee, in many cases, is used to offset increasing costs as one might be required to move from independent living to assisted, medical, or memory care.

CCRCs may offer one or all three of the following contracts:

- **Life Care:** Most expensive option but covers even the most expensive services without increasing the fees.
- **Modified Contract:** Offers certain services for a set period and then, if additional services are needed, the fees increase.

- **Fee for Service:** Assisted-living, skilled nursing, and memory care services are an increased fee.

An advantage of providing several levels of care means your elder can age in one place. Moving from place to place becomes increasingly difficult as we age.

If you are looking at a CCRC with your elder, make sure the CCRC provides full financial disclosure and remember to ask for formal audits. If the CCRC does require a high buy-in and is not financially solvent (or may not be in the near future), your elder could lose her entire savings. Also, whether you select a CCRC or an ALF, ask if your elder can visit for a weekend. Many will provide this opportunity.

Considerations for Your Elder to Ponder

- I prefer to live in one place for the rest of my life regardless of illness and needs.
- If the CCRC requires a high buy-in, I can afford that buy-in and feel this is a good use of retirement funds.
- I prefer to live in a larger environment than adult foster care.

More Information

AARP on "What Is a Continuing Care Retirement Community?" http://www.aarp.org/relationships/caregiving-resource-center/info-09-2010/ho_continuing_care_retirement_communities.html
On CCRC accreditation: http://www.carf.org/home/
USA Today **article on CCRCs:** http://www.usatoday.com/story/money/columnist/powell/2014/10/18/continuing-care-independent-living-assisted-living-powell/17447609/
Book: *What's the Deal with Retirement Communities?* by Brad C. Breeding, Certified Financial Planner. Available on Amazon.com and at other bookstores.

For a form to use for keeping track of addresses, phone numbers, e-mail addresses, first impressions, and the like, of **"Potential CCRCs,"** go to https://rowman.com/ISBN/9781442265462.

ASSISTED LIVING FACILITIES

ALFs encompass a broad range of living styles—from independent living in small cottage homes or apartments to "full-care" living including skilled nursing or memory care. Some facilities focus on a specific level or type of support such as memory care. In general, assisted living facilities can be identified by the following characteristics:

- Typically, twenty or more (could be several hundred) elders living together.
- Most offer increasing levels of custodial or medical care.
- For active elders, many offer options for group activities and trips.
- Great for people who like to be around a lot of other people.
- Can be less expensive than twenty-four/seven "equal" home health care, given home care is $20–$25/hour for nonmedical care.
- More expensive than adult foster care.
- Services are "á la carte" and, as the elder needs more help, the costs increase.
- Most are transparent about telling prospective residents what the costs of all care levels will be.
- Prior to admittance, the elder is evaluated during an "intake session" to determine where she fits and the cost of the care.

Due Diligence

When you are comparing different assisted living facilities, be diligent about *understanding the costs and how they escalate with advanced care*. What are all the exact fees? For example, although not as common as with CCRCs, some ALFs charge a buy-in fee. You might also need to make a deposit. What are the monthly fees? They can be anywhere from $3,000 to $7,000—or even higher. If your elder suffers increasing disability and illness, are there escalating fees? Also, be clear on any refundable deposit fees or buy-in costs if your elder moves to a different home or dies.

During visits, be sure to ask about the *financial viability of the facility, staff turnover rates, and if there are any complaints filed with the ombudsman* (and the outcomes). Then call your ombudsman to make sure the facility is forthcoming. Check out this link to find the ombudsman in your area: http://theconsumervoice.org/get_help.

Want to Know More?

AARP on "Assisted Living—What to Ask": http://assets.aarp.org/external _sites/caregiving/options/assisted_living.html

Assisted Living Federation of America (ALFA): A great site for general information about assisted living including what to expect and some of the options for assisted care; also offers a satisfaction survey of assisted living facilities; http://www.alfa.org/alfa/default.asp

Federal government fact sheet on assisted living: http://www.eldercare.gov/
  Eldercare.NET/Public/Resources/Factsheets/Assisted_Living.aspx
Questions to ask when you visit assisted living facilities: http://www.aplace
  formom.com/senior-care-resources/articles/assisted-living-residence-
  checklist

IS ASSISTED CARE THE
ANSWER FOR YOUR ELDER?

Some people choose to age at home for as long as they can manage, and
then they may move to an assisted care facility. Other people move before they need added support, because they feel safer, enjoy being surrounded by many other people, and they want to participate in the activities
offered.

If your elder is considering assisted care living, join her in visiting and
comparing several facilities. Discussing her answers to these questions might
help your elder determine if assisted care will be a good fit:

• Would you enjoy living in a larger facility with a lot of residents, staff, and
  activities (or would you prefer a smaller place with only a few older adults
  such as an adult foster care home)?
• Would you enjoy and participate in arranged outings and in the activities
  at the facility?
• Do you want to be in a place where you live independently as long as
  possible and also have other levels of service available as you age such as
  custodial care, healthcare services, medical care wing, and memory care
  wing, if needed?
• Is the facility inviting and safe (smell, light, universal design features,
  etc.)?
• Is the room large enough for you?
• If you own a pet, can the pet come with you?
• If you run out of resources, will the facility accept Medicaid? If not, what
  transition plan does the facility offer?
• Is the facility licensed and is the license up to date?
• Are there complaints about the facility? If yes, what are they? Contact your
  state ombudsman to learn more about each facility.

Once your elder has answered these questions and discussed her answers
with you, explore finishing this phrase: "Assisted care living seems right or
wrong for me because _____."

SELECTING AN ASSISTED LIVING FACILITY

Moving from one's home is a big decision and should be made carefully. Visit several facilities and stop by more than once with your elder. Maybe she can spend the weekend. Ask if you and your elder can have lunch and see if she likes the food and whether the people in the dining room are enjoying their meal. Keep a chart of first impressions, so you can compare apples to apples. You may want to review these questions with your elder after a visit to each potential ALF:

- Does it feel comfortable? Can it eventually feel "like home"?
- Is it inviting and safe (smell, light, universal design features, etc.)?
- Do the residents and staff seem happy?
- Does its location meet your needs for connection with friends, family, and other contacts such as your doctors?
- Is transportation available so you can go on personal outings (appointments such as medical and hair, shopping, religious services, the movies, and the like)?
- Is transportation limited to facility-planned group outings?
- Is it important that you are able to spend time outside? If so, does the facility have walking areas?
- Can visitors drop by during reasonable hours without making prior arrangements with the staff? If not, why not?
- Can you have your own selection of food in your room?
- Can you prepare meals in your room? Is this important to you?
- Is the food prepared by the facility nutritious and appetizing?
- Can the facility support your current or future needs for medical and custodial care?
- Are there illnesses, diseases, or other changes that could cause the facility to require you to leave?
- If you are on Medicaid, will the facility ask you to leave if its policy of accepting Medicaid changes?
- Does it provide a statement of care and describe its philosophy?
- Are pets welcomed? This may be a positive or a negative for you.
- If you are LGBT, will you feel welcome?
- Is there a gym, pool, or exercise program so you can continue to stay active if you are able?

For a form to use for keeping track of addresses, phone numbers, e-mail addresses, first impressions, and the like, of **"Potential Assisted Living Facilities,"** go to https://rowman.com/ISBN/9781442265462.

MEMORY CARE FACILITIES

As noted, many ALFs and CCRCs provide dedicated units or rooms for memory care. However, there are also "stand-alone" memory care facilities. (See our "Medical" section for information on dementia and other mental health issues.)

Both stand-alone memory care facilities and memory care units within ALFs and CCRCs pay close attention to structural design—creating rooms, hallways, and common areas that are safe and visually supportive but not confusing and overwhelming to the elder suffering cognitive challenges. Memory care facilities also focus on building extra safety features, preventing elders from wandering away from the facility. In addition, they often require specialized staff training. With the more intense hands-on care, extra security features, and specialized training, memory care facilities are more expensive than assisted care living.

To decide if your elder needs memory care, explore the following statements:

• I feel my parent is no longer safe where she is currently living.
• I prefer a stand-alone memory care facility.
• I prefer memory care provided within an ALF or CCRC.

Resources

Assisted Living Federation of America (ALFA): Memory care is addressed on this web page; http://www.alfa.org/News/2306/The-Memory-Care-Opportunity

Alzheimer's Organization on "When Living at Home Is No Longer an Option": http://www.alz.org/care/alzheimers-dementia-residential-facilities.asp#when

Federal State and County Resources: This highly recommended web page can help you locate many state and county resources on aging. 1-800-677-1116, http://www.eldercare.gov/Eldercare.NET/Public/Index.aspx

LeadingAge Center for Aging Services Technology (CAST): A resource of contacts for many elder services and needs; http://www.leadingage.org/FindMember.aspx

What Is Memory Care and Where Can I Find It? http://www.aplaceformom.com/alzheimers-care

For a form to use for keeping track of addresses, phone numbers, e-mail addresses, first impressions, and the like, of **"Potential Memory Care Facilities,"** go to https://rowman.com/ISBN/9781442265462.

SOCIAL PILLAR OF AGING WELLBEING

Humankind has not woven the web of life. We are but one thread within it. Whatever we do to the web, we do to ourselves. All things are bound together. All things connect.

—Chief Seattle, 1854

Chapter Four

MARY JO'S FIRESIDE CHAT

Social Strategy: Don't Worry! Be Happy! How Does an Elder Find Meaning and Joy Despite So Much Loss?

As we slip over the threshold of age sixty, we begin to notice more substantial changes in our bodies. Energy changes, mobility is more difficult, and even memory slows. Up until then, we may have had changes in vision and hearing and some aches and pains, but soon we start hearing about friends becoming seriously ill or dying and our own experience can shift into new territory of threatening limitations. By ages seventy-five to eighty, days can be filled with loss. For many, having to give up their driver's license is a profound change and usually a big point of contention with family members. Incontinence may limit our ability to leave home. Dear ones in our lives may be dying, and, growing into the oldest old, we can be forced to say good-bye to siblings and even children who die.

An elder's world can shrink very quickly. Many slip into depression with no understanding of how to create a present that brings them satisfaction and wellbeing. Pain, illness, and financial issues—all can conspire to keep an elder down and unable to help himself. This is the time when you as the caregiver can provide opportunities for your elder to find new ways of experiencing the world.

During my assessment of an elder's profile and condition, what I consider to be one of the most important areas on which to focus is understanding what has brought meaning to that person throughout his life. What wishes does he have for his day-to-day living? Almost always the oldest old elders ask me, "Why am I still here?" They quickly follow this question with, "I do not want to be a burden to my family." This is where our society has relegated elders to feeling as though they are nothing more than a bother. It is difficult for them to dream or imagine a different way of being if this is their starting point.

All too often in our culture, if you are not producing resources instead of consuming them, you are perceived as worthless, which results in too many elders today suffering from loneliness, boredom, and depression. Dr. Bill Thomas has been an important advocate, along with his wife, Jude, in addressing this epidemic. Through their dedication to quality eldercare and the development of the elder-centered care homes based on their "Eden philosophy," they have remapped how nursing homes and memory care homes can function in America to address these issues.

For aging in place, there have been multiple studies about living healthy and staying engaged. *National Geographic* explorer Dan Buettner, in his wonderful book, *The Blue Zones: Lessons for Living Longer from the People Who've Lived the Longest,* says that "a long, healthy life is no accident. It begins with good genes, but it also depends on good habits." That is, if you adopt the right lifestyle, chances are you may live up to a decade longer. So what's the magic formula for success?

To find the answer, Buettner led a team of researchers across the globe to uncover the secrets of "blue zones"—geographic regions where high percentages of centenarians are enjoying remarkably long, full lives. They found that the recipe for longevity is deeply intertwined with community, lifestyle, and spirituality. Feeling a sense of purpose, being valued, and having a reason to get up in the morning are some of the things "blue zone" elders share. Buettner writes, "You won't find longevity in a bottle of diet pills or with hormone therapy. You'll find it by embracing a few simple but powerful habits, and by creating the right community around yourself."

One of my favorite elders, Stewart, is a ninety-year-old man confined to a wheelchair. Stewart has five devoted sons who work hard as a team to ensure that Stewart has a good quality of life. They have a great philosophy of respecting Stewart's abilities to do what he can until he can't. Although they get along great, the sons often trip over each other trying to provide the best for their dad. They called me to do an integrative life assessment and provide a care plan so they could each have their own tasks to help manage.

Stewart lives in his own condo with a caregiver, watches sports on TV, and manages some of his investments, although one of his sons shares access to his finances to keep an eye on activities. After spending a few hours with Stewart and one of his sons, I identified a few gaps in Stewart's care, but, just as important, I could see where he could use additional companionship from elders in his age group. His family was very attentive with visits and involved him in family events, in addition to managing his care, but the isolation of being at home alone prevented him from interacting with other elders.

The sons quickly activated the care plan and put it into effect to create support strategies for appropriate activities. Stewart and his sons made a clear choice of quality over quantity. He wants his life to be interesting and involved. He was fortunate enough to have a family who felt the same way.

In this "Social" section of *Eldercare 101*, Susan Cain McCarty shares some of the social challenges our elders face in living fully and staying engaged until the end. As noted in the "Living Environment" section, Susan is an ALCM, certified senior advisor, and gerontologist. She has a deep interest in elders' stories and what brings meaning to their lives. She is especially interested in the oldest old, those over eighty-five who often have limited mobility and are in decline. I have asked her also to share her strategies for a major issue many caregivers face: elders driving a car. In addition, she provides many resources, technology aids, and insights about strategies to keep elders engaged in their lives and yours.

Social Considerations

Susan Cain McCarty, MAIS, CSA

Although deciding where to live is critical and occupies the minds of many elders, there are many other important topics and issues elders need to address—such as how to facilitate downsizing and physically moving, driving or not, and keeping yourself safe from scams. This section will touch on these issues and more.

LIFE REIMAGINED

TEN TIPS FOR FINDING MEANING OR PURPOSE IN LIFE

As we retire, our families grow up and need us less, and we lose many loved ones and friends. These losses (sometimes coupled with a loss of independence or financial freedom) leave many elders struggling to find meaning and purpose in life, which, ultimately, affects their ability to live fully and joyfully. However, life in one's seventies, eighties, and nineties *can* still be full of meaning! In fact, research shows that those who have a sense of purpose also have a lower incidence of illness including stroke. In essence, finding or redefining your purpose can give you a longer lease on life.

This tip list is intended to inspire your elder to think about how to rediscover or redefine life's purpose right now. Maybe it's time to take up a new hobby, enjoy helping others, or adapt to new limitations.

1. **Cultivate spirituality:** We often mistake spirituality for religion. While spirituality may be tied to religion, for many or even most, it's that deep inward sense of purpose and meaning. For some, spirituality exists within us in the form of a gift or talent such as music, singing, writing, baking, or sewing. Or you may find spirituality in the beauty of deep thought, meditation, prayer, or maybe walking a labyrinth. No one definition of spirituality exists because we each define it by that which is deep inside. Some people find a place of worship where they can cultivate spirituality with others who practice their spirituality in a similar way. Others engage in-home spiritual practitioners. For further exploration, be sure to read our "Spiritual" section at the end of this book. You also might want to check out this article on cultivating your spiritual side: http://www.redbookmag. com/health-wellness/advice/life-changes-spiritual-tips.

2. **Volunteer:** Who needs help in your community and how can you help them? Your elder could help at schools, children's daycare centers, or hospitals; spend time at the local food bank straightening shelves; or make and deliver a meal once a week for a friend or a person in need. Is he an animal lover? Pet shelters always are looking for volunteers. Perhaps getting out is difficult, but your elder could make calls to others who are homebound. Ask your local place of worship for a list of people who might enjoy a phone call (or an in-person visit if your elder is capable of visiting). If your elder is homebound, you might use the same method to find a companion for him. There are also a number of online organizations that match volunteers to a need. Check out **Volunteer Match** (http://www.volunteermatch .org) and **Create the Good** (http://www.createthegood.org).

3. **Take a class:** Much of our lives we wish we had time to study something new. Now's your elder's chance! He might learn a foreign language online or take an art history class at the local junior college. Also, many universities offer free or reduced tuition classes for elders.

4. **Write his life story:** Encourage your elder to start anywhere (who are you now, who were you at age eight, what was your first job, etc.). If that seems daunting, have him try working with a certified guided autobiographer (contact Anita Reyes at anitareyes@cox.net and ask if she knows of someone in your area) or a personal historian (check out the Association of Personal Historians at http://www.personalhistorians.org). If your elder can't write, consider video or tape recording his life story or telling it to someone else who will record it. This is such a wonderful legacy gift for family and friends. Most elders who take the time to share their story find joy in the experience. Maybe you can even have it published for your elder.

5. **Write or record a cookbook** of favorite recipes and those of relatives and friends (be sure to give them credit) or explore the family genealogy. Perhaps even suggest to your elder that he combine genealogy and recipes and share the finished product with the family.

6. **Enjoy reading?** Have your elder try a challenging book or author. If he can't see well enough to read, check out audiobooks through your local library, iTunes, Amazon.com, and other online book distributors. Maybe he can even join (or start!) a book group and discuss what he is reading. Contact your local library to find out about its monthly book groups; some are genre based. That is, maybe you can find a group that reads and discusses just mysteries. The options are endless. Libraries are also great places to volunteer!

7. **Does your elder enjoy board games or card games** but not have a partner? Check with the local senior center, parks and recreation programs, and adult daycare centers to see if you can find a game partner for your elder. There are also many games online.

8. **How about brain teasers to help improve memory?** Lumosity.com is popular and good for keeping your brain well exercised; however, there are many online brain teaser sites, so search online for "brain teaser." Show your elder how to access the websites and do the exercises.

9. **Think of other hobbies** once enjoyed but given up. Maybe your elder would like to join a choir or a local orchestra. Perhaps there were hobbies he always wanted to try and didn't such as building models or painting. If your elder is homebound, you might look for card groups or chess clubs in your area that may come to your elder's residence. Also, check out this website for more ideas about hobbies for the elderly: https://myage ingparent.com/life/health-life/best-activities-and-hobbies-for-your-older-parent.

10. **If you have a loved one with dementia or Alzheimer's disease**, meaning is found in new ways. Consider art therapy, music therapy, and, if he has a religious affiliation, perhaps a prayer circle where the rhythm of the prayers is often still encoded in advanced memory loss.

More Resources

A Good Read: *Living with Purpose in a Worn-Out Body: Spiritual Encouragement for Older Adults* by Missy Buchanan; http://www.amazon.com/Living-Purpose-Worn-Out-Body-Encouragement/dp/083589942X

AARP online program to "Help Make Dreams Become Reality": https://lifereimagined.aarp.org/

THE IMPORTANCE OF COMMUNICATION AND CONNECTION WITH A SUPPORTIVE VILLAGE

Talking and sharing are perhaps the best therapy for everyone at any age. However, as we become older and suffer losses, we may become less mobile and have fewer opportunities to interact with others. Whether you live near your elders or far away, know that communicating with others regularly is important! You may want to develop a formal plan for helping your elders to keep loved ones, friends, and extended community in their lives—both for social interaction and for medical or health support. Sometimes, an elder peer counselor, available through regional programs, might keep your elder on a "social" track. You can find elder peer counselors in your area by searching online for "elder or senior peer counselor [and your city]" or by asking an ALCM to connect with one.

Community Resources for Staying Connected When Your Elder Is Mobile

- **Faith community.** A person's place of worship also can be a place of companionship.
- **Senior center.** At senior centers, elders often can find others with similar interests—from pickleball to pool to bridge.
- **Exercise facility/gym.** Many community centers and gyms have exercise classes specifically geared for the elderly. If your elder is mobile, he can get exercise—as well as social interaction—at the gym.
- **Local library.** Most libraries welcome the elderly as volunteers; your elder can make a host of new friends there.
- **Local college.** Many local colleges offer classes to the elderly for free or at reduced rates. College is a great place to make friends—at any age.

Community Resources for Staying Connected When Your Elder Is Not Mobile

- **Faith community.** Let your elder's pastor, minister, imam, or rabbi know your elder would appreciate visits or having someone come to share rituals or sacraments.
- **Senior center.** Mobile elders often volunteer to visit those who are homebound.
- **Local library.** Many libraries offer a free service of mailing large-print books, books on CD, magazines, movies, and more to residents who are physically unable to visit their local library.

Connecting through Technology

- **Caringbridge.org** allows you to set up a site where plans can be made for food delivery, visiting, or taking an elder to the doctor. This site also has a guestbook where those who are invited into this "caring community" can leave comments. This site is supportive of the tough challenge of long-distance care giving.
- You can set up an **informal newsletter** that can be shared on Google Plus or another sharing site so everyone can add comments and pictures. Another option: You can circulate the newsletter through e-mail, and each person can contribute and pass it on to the next.
- While communicating through computers, tablets, and phone calls can't take the place of personal touch and interaction, **video chats** can extend the reach of your elder to other loved ones, allowing him to "see" people

and share more fully than through phone calls. Products include FaceTime, Skype, Firefox Hello, Facebook Chat, ooVoo, and many others.
- On some days, an in-person visit is critical, and on other days your elder may be content to be updated through **social networking products** such as Facebook, Instagram, LinkedIn, Pinterest, Yahoo, and other social sites. Teach your elder how to use at least one of these sites. If he has a smartphone, he may want to use the app that corresponds to the site, allowing him to post comments and photos while on the go. For example, your elder might post notes, photos, and links about how he is doing and about issues he finds interesting, connecting with people and communities important to him. Be sure to alert your elder that everything on these sites can be available to anyone unless you lock down the information. Each site is different regarding how you can protect your pictures and postings, so research each site carefully.

> To download a **"My Village"** form for keeping track of names, addresses, phone numbers, and e-mail addresses of friends, family members, neighbors, etc., in your elder's life, go to https://rowman.com/ISBN/9781442265462.

FIVE WAYS OF *BEING* TOGETHER WITH YOUR ELDER

1. **Table Talk: The Beauty of Eating Meals Together.** Spending time around the family table has been proven to stave off teenage delinquency, increase an adolescent's sense of self-identity, and improve SAT scores. But the benefits of "table talk" are not limited to one generation! Eating together as a family creates a sense of purpose and belonging that can nurture everyone—including elders. Studies show, even in the most dysfunctional families, the benefit of eating dinner around the table has profound and lasting, positive effects on every member. For example, when grandparents are at the table, they share gifts of wisdom and teach their families how to age, how to live, and how to love.

    Well-known geriatrician Dr. Bill Thomas has taken this research and used it to advance family-style meals in retirement communities and nursing homes. In fact, he uses the "table" as the centerpiece to his Green House living environments to fight depression, boredom, and loneliness in elders. See the Eden Alternative at http://www.EdenAlt.org for more information on an Eden Alternative community in your area.
2. **Memory Gardens.** Do some research to find out if a memory garden exists in your area. If your elder lives at home or in a facility, consider building a memory garden with him. This is a place of beauty where Dad

can touch and feel the plants and flowers; where he can plant and play; where can simply sit and *be* with the smells, sounds, colors, and sensations feeding his senses—and his soul.

3. **Music Therapy.** With dementia, music memories are often the very last to be affected by degenerative disease. An exciting new discovery has been made using iPods with elders suffering with dementias. Using music therapy, some people "come back to life," after even years of silence. Visit http://musicandmemory.org/ for more information. The doctors behind this work have been featured in an inspirational documentary called, *Alive Inside*. Be prepared to be inspired as you watch the trailer available at http://www.aliveinside.us/#trailer.

4. **Art Therapy.** A longstanding tradition of mixing art and psychotherapy enables elders to create and explore their inner landscape without words. Art therapy professionals offer programs that can provide a new meaning and richness specifically for elders living with dementia—and their loved ones. Find an art therapist in your area at http://arttherapy.org. Also, the Alzheimer's Association has auctions around the country called Memories in Art that feature works of art created by people with Alzheimer's disease. See http://www.alz.org.

There's an App for That!

Check out **Computer Art Therapy**. This app allows elders to create art without needing expensive supplies.

---

5. **Storytelling.** Elders have a need to tell their stories. Doing so is a way to process and make sense of their lives as they see their lives transitioning. For individuals with dementia, the long-term memory center of their brain is often one of the last parts of the brain to be affected. Telling their stories is a valuable way to pass on wisdom and family genealogy to the next generation. Who knows what you will discover? There are many emerging ways to capture your elder's stories and history with photos, videos, writing, and guided interviews. Stories can be recorded through traditional methods or in podcasts; old photos and films can be recreated through digital transfer. For a professional feel, you can hire a personal historian to help your elder tell his life story: http://www.personalhistorians.org. For more on creating life stories, search the Internet for terms such as "creating life story," "legacy," "genealogy," and "elder life stories." Also check out commercial support for creating legacy books and videos at companies such as http://www.timelines-inc.com.

> **There's an App for That!**
>
> **Ancestory.com** and **Family Tree Maker** are two of many genealogy apps that also allow photos and stories to be captured.

ADULT DAY CARE

Sometimes the activities at home just don't offer enough social, emotional, physical, or mental stimulation. Sometimes a partner just needs time alone. There are many reasons why elders opt to participate in "adult day care." Here are some need-to-know facts about adult daycare facilities:

- Provide drop-in activities for elders in a safe environment.
- Typically open during daytime hours on Monday through Friday.
- Usually feature dining as well as art and craftmaking, music, and other forms of entertainment and enrichment.
- Some offer day trips.
- Some provide transportation (i.e., "pickup and delivery").
- Some offer health and medical services.
- Some serve elders with Alzheimer's disease and dementia.

Adult day care is a great option if one partner is taking care of the other and one needs some "alone time." By one partner going to adult day care once a week or more, the other has time for his or her own needs and interests.

If an elder is being treated medically while at these facilities, part or most of the cost may be covered by Medicare, Medicaid, or LTC insurances. This is not always the case, however, so it pays to check into this carefully.

Details, Details!

Eldercare Fact Sheet about Adult Day Care: http://www.eldercare.gov/ Eldercare.NET/Public/Resources/Factsheets/Adult_Day_Care.aspx

Eldercare Locator: To find services in your state and county, call 1-800-677-1116 or check out http://www.eldercare.gov.

> To download a form for keeping track of names, addresses, phone numbers, and e-mail addresses of **"Potential Adult Daycare Programs,"** go to https:// rowman.com/ISBN/9781442265462.

TRANSPORTATION ISSUES

SHOULD YOUR ELDER BE DRIVING?

We all value our independence. In fact, when asking elders about what's important as they age, "independence" is usually second or third—following health and having enough money to pay for retirement years.

Most of us are accustomed to running errands any time the mood strikes. But given that many elders will live into their eighties, nineties, and even up to one hundred, most will give up their license and car at some point. Knowing when to give up driving and then researching and planning how to still be independent without a car are key steps for elders. See the many resources on the following pages.

Frequently, many elders believe their relatives and friends are too quick to suggest they give up their license. In reality, the relatives and friends can objectively judge their loved one's driving skills. Here are a few questions to have your elder ask himself as a way to reflect upon whether he should still be driving. If there are more "yes" answers (or even a few), suggest that your elder participate in a more rigorous self-rating (see the AAA link under "Be Sure! Be Safe! Resources") or take a driver safety course; check out the AARP website link to find one in his neighborhood.

- When you are frustrated or anxious, does it affect your driving?
- Have you experienced situations where your reaction time slowed to the point where you put yourself or others in danger?
- Do you misjudge distances between cars and rate of speed so that you might be a danger when merging into traffic?
- Do you take medications that affect your driving? (If you aren't sure, talk with your doctor and pharmacist and follow up every time a medication is changed.)
- Have you dozed off at a stop sign or light?
- Have your family and friends expressed concern about your driving?
- Have you been pulled over, received tickets, or had minor or major accidents over the past few years?
- Do you struggle to remember how to get to locations you have frequented in the past or even get lost?
- Does your vision impact your ability to read road signs, road markings, and traffic signals?
- When driving, do you ever find you have forgotten where you are going?
- Do you struggle more with nighttime driving?
- Do you struggle with freeway driving?
- Do you struggle driving in new, unfamiliar places?

After reviewing the previous questions with your elder, ask: What do you honestly think? Should you turn over your keys or not?

Driver Safety Resources

This is a matter of life and death—your elder's and someone else's.

AAA's Self-Rating Tool to Help You Determine If You're a Safe Driver: This AAA brochure, "Drivers 65 Plus," features a fifteen-question self-rating driving assessment exercise designed to help you examine your driving performance; http://seniordriving.aaa.com/evaluate-your-driving-ability/self-rating-tool

AARP on "When It's Time to Stop Driving": http://www.aarp.org/home-garden/transportation/info-05-2010/Warning_Signs_Stopping.html

AARP Safe Driver Course: For online classes, go to http://www.aarpdriversafety.org. To find driver safety classroom courses in your area, check out http://www.aarp.org/applications/VMISLocator/searchDspLocations.action.

American Occupational Therapy Association (AOTA) Perspective on Driving and Mobility: Occupational therapy practitioners have the science-based knowledge to understand progressive conditions and life changes that can affect driving. On this web page, AOTA offers tools to help individuals make a smoother transition from driving to using other forms of transportation. In doing so, they help people maintain their autonomy, independence, and sense of worth. Check out both these links: http://www.aota.org/older driver and http://www.aota.org/About-Occupational-Therapy/Patients-Clients/Adults/OlderDrivers/DrivingSafelyAsYouAge.aspx.

Federal Government's Fact Sheet on How to Talk with an Older Driver about Concerns: http://www.eldercare.gov/Eldercare.NET/Public/Resources/Factsheets/Talk_Elder_Driver.aspx

Liberty Mutual's Safe Driving Tips for Elders: http://www.libertymutual.com/auto-insurance/senior-driving/studies/safety-tips

Take an Actual Driver's Test . . . and Reevaluate Often

If the self-rated tools or questionnaires above raise any red flags for your elder, he should seriously consider paying for a driver's test in his car. Being tested by a professional is the most realistic assessment of driving ability. To find professionals who offer private driver's tests, search online for "private driving test [your town/city]."

Also, if your elder has been tested and given the green light for now, reevaluate every six to twelve months. There also is the option of suggesting "in-between" restrictions such as: don't drive (1) at night, (2) on the freeway, and (3) in new, unfamiliar places.

HIGH-TECH DRIVING GADGETS

Improve Driving Habits

Installed into cars, these products collect information about driving behaviors. If drivers "score well," consumers are rewarded with lower insurance rates. One company boasts discounts of up to 30 percent. Note: The providers claim the results will not hurt the rates. As of the printing of this book, products include **Drivewise from Allstate**, **Drive Safe and Save from State Farm**, and **Snapshot from Progressive**.

These products and offerings aren't available in all states. If your elder doesn't have insurance with these providers, check with his insurer as others will likely follow suit and provide similar products. Also, search your app store for the terms "driving," "driving skills," and "driving simulator." You can even find an app for many state-driving laws. One app to measure driving behavior is **Driving Curve** for iPhone and Android.

Find the Car

At any age, we sometimes forget where we parked our car. Today, however, you can find your car with a phone app. A few popular apps include **Find My Car**, **Find My Car Smarter**, and **My Car Locator**. Some of these apps will track your car to a general location, whereas others can take you to a specific spot within a large parking lot or garage. Some products require both an app and a device installed in the car itself; others only require downloading the app. Apps of any type increase in number daily, so do a search for "find my car" through iTunes, your mobile phone provider store, or on the Internet.

Everything about the Car

Although somewhat expensive, **Zubie** works like a fitness tracker for a car. This small device plugs into a diagnostics port under a car's dashboard and syncs to a smartphone app that keeps tabs on the location of a vehicle as well as its health (e.g., gas-price and mileage tracker, battery and engine monitor, driving habits such as sudden stopping and excessive speeding). As an invited user, you can follow your elder's car—helping to keep tabs on if the "check engine" light stays on for weeks. See http://www.zubie.com for details.

CAREGIVER CHALLENGE: TAKING AWAY THE KEYS

Our cars often become integral to our sense of independence, and our independence is tied to self-esteem, even to our sense of purpose. Telling an elder he must stop driving is painful. If you need to do so, because his driving has become poor, you will want to enlist support from other family members, your elder's doctor, and even friends in law enforcement. The idea isn't to "gang up" on your elder but to help him see the reality of the dangers of driving, as an elder's reflexes and cognitive ability slow down. Also, keep in mind that, when elders turn over the keys, they must have accessible and affordable transportation alternatives. Without the ability to be active in the community, elders can become homebound and depressed and will often age more quickly than those still driving.

What Does That Difficult Conversation Look Like?

- First, begin the conversation with your elder far, far in advance of the need. That way you can both agree to conditions around making the decision. This may not change that he becomes upset, but you will have a plan.
- Anticipate that, no matter how well orchestrated the discussion, your elder will be upset and even angry.
- Be empathetic and respectful. Use language that doesn't make your elder feel as if you are the parent and he is a child. Ask questions about his thoughts, ideas, and feelings.
- Talk about "why": medical changes in hearing, sight, reaction time, cognitive changes, as well as his safety and that of others. You may point to articles about people who have been hurt in accidents caused by an elder's slow reaction time or pressing the gas instead of the brake, which is actually common, particularly in parking lots.
- Propose plans and programs for how he can maintain an active life without driving.
- If you've witnessed events that cause you to believe it's time for the elder to stop driving, talk with the elder's doctor. The doctor cannot share information with you about what he has witnessed about the elder unless you have POA. Laws and regulations concerning a doctor's responsibility vary from state to state. In some states, doctors are legally bound to report concerns to the Department of Motor Vehicles (DMV) about an elder's ability to drive safely. Many states also provide physicians with immunity from litigation for reporting an incapacitated elder driver. Regardless of your state laws, competent physicians are concerned for your elder's safety and the safety of others on the road, and sharing your thoughts with them is important for everyone's safety.
- Suggest that your elder speak with his doctor (or attorney) openly and honestly; be sure to have spoken first with the professional so he can see the "other story" to what your elder may share.

- Your elder may be concerned about his driver's license being his primary identification card. Explain that the DMV will provide a standard ID card, and offer to drive him to the DMV to apply for and acquire the new card.
- Avoid forcefully taking the keys or car from your elder. For some adult children, however, that does happen. For more on how to legally stop an elder from driving, see: http://www.agingcare.com/Articles/Ways-to-Legally-Get-Your-Elderly-Parent-s-Keys-112307.htm.
- Some states have established procedures for voluntary reporting of unsafe drivers. Nonmandatory reports come from law enforcement officers, physicians and other medical providers, family members, social service providers, courts, DMV office employees, and others. Although most states do not accept anonymous reports, the reporters are immune from civil liability. Based on the information contained in the report, a person's license may be immediately suspended or the person may be given an amount of time to submit additional medical information or pass DMV tests before a suspension action is taken. DMV will notify the person by mail of any actions that must be taken to keep or regain his license. To learn about your state's unsafe driver programs, search online for "DMV unsafe driver [your state]."

Also Check Out

Help Guide on "How Aging Affects Driving" and "When Is It Time to Stop Driving": A great resource with lots of questions and answers including "How to Talk to Loved Ones About Driving Concerns," http://www.helpguide.org/articles/aging-well/age-and-driving-safety-tips.htm

TRANSPORTATION ALTERNATIVES

If your elder gives up the keys to the car, have a plan in place for alternative transportation options. Transportation for elders is generally offered as:

- Individual door-to-door service
- Fixed route with scheduled services
- Ridesharing with volunteer drivers
- Family and friends

Because transportation options are specific to communities, begin your search for options with your local Area Agency on Aging. Also ask your local faith community if volunteer transportation services are available; sometimes these options are free or inexpensive.

Ready Resources

Area Agency on Aging (AAA): Find your state AAA, then contact the state agency to find your county resources; http://www.aoa.gov/AoA_programs/ OAA/How_To_Find/Agencies/find_agencies.aspx.

Federal Government Eldercare Locator: http://www.eldercare.gov

Helpguide on Knowing Your Transportation Alternatives: http://www.help guide.org/articles/aging-well/age-and-driving-safety-tips.htm

National Center on Senior Transportation: http://www.seniortransporta tion.net/

National Transit Hotline: Can provide the names of local transit providers who receive federal money to provide transportation to the elderly and people with disabilities. Call Toll Free 1-800-527-8279.

For a downloadable form to keep track of **"My Possible Rides,"** go to https:// rowman.com/ISBN/9781442265462.

MANAGING A MOVE

NOTES ON MOVING: THE ELDER, THE STUFF, AND THE BELOVED PET

Maybe your elder is ready to move and eager to clear out the extra "stuff" in the house, attic, and garage. Or perhaps he must move because of finances or health concerns—and it's not his first choice. Whether your elder perceives the move as positive or negative, it's still stressful emotionally and physically. There's even a medical diagnosis for this stress: relocation stress syndrome (RSS). Symptoms can include anxiety, trouble sleeping, feeling exhausted even when you do sleep well, and overeating or undereating. A sense of deep sadness and the grief that comes with loss also often accompany moving. If the elder is suffering from cognitive disorder or physical challenges, RSS will likely increase significantly.

Like most big changes in life—even when it's desired change—there is a grieving process and there's no shortcut. The predictable steps are denial, anger, bargaining, depression, and acceptance. Few march straight through the process; most will bounce among all the feelings for a while. For more on this process, check out books and articles by Elizabeth Kübler-Ross or go to PsychCentral at http://psychcentral.com/lib/the-5-stages-of-loss-and-grief/000617.

Here are a few tips and resources that may help elders when they move:

The Elder

- First and foremost, if the elder is capable and interested in participating, include him in all decisions. As you get embroiled in the process, regularly ask yourself if you are making decisions alone that should include the elder.
- As much as possible, keep meds, meals, rest, and exercise schedules regular.
- Create a few "go ahead" boxes or plastic tubs that stay with the elder until he moves into the new home. One of the boxes will include personal items, toiletries, clothing, bedding, and books the elder will need right away upon resettling. Also create a similar box for the new home that includes cleaning supplies, paper towels, toilet paper, hand soap, towels, and the like. This allows the elder to move in and feel comfortable he has "necessities" until all the other items arrive and are unpacked.
- Determine the move schedule and where the elder will be day by day and share this schedule.
- Allow time to process this life-altering event. Talk through what's exciting about the move and what's causing distress. Most of the time, listening is more important than providing answers.
- Have the new home set up before the elder enters the first time (unless he wants to be actively involved in the unpacking) and make sure treasured items are prominently placed.
- For the first few weeks, help the elder adjust by spending more time with him. Consider a regular time at lunch or dinner, because eating with strangers or alone in a new apartment can be daunting.

If you have the resources, consider hiring a senior move manager or ALCM to help plan, find the best resources, and execute the move. Locate senior move managers at http://www.nasmm.org and ALCMs at http://www.aginglifecare.org.

The "Stuff"

- Look through the house and make a list of items that seem to be most important to the elder (e.g., photo albums, a few knick-knacks, framed

artwork, an afghan knitted by a loved one, that favorite chair and lamp for reading, and, of course, the books kept and reread year after year).
- Measure each room in the new home and draw in the big pieces of furniture. Then talk about what will fit and what won't.
- If adult children or friends are keeping items for the elder, make sure the elder knows where and how those items are housed.
- Don't forget to save holiday decorations that have meant a great deal year after year and bring those in at the appropriate times.
- Eat up! Plan creative meals, allowing the elder to use up most of the food in the freezer, fridge, and pantry. If there is still food left over, consider donating it to a shelter.
- Have large bins for keep, recycle, trash, and toxins. Purchase a box of large, heavy-duty trash bags; as you move room by room, you can collect the trash easily.
- Consider whether an estate sale is the best way to re-home items that won't fit or aren't needed—or whether you want to donate to a charity (and get a tax write-off).
- Cut costs wherever possible to cover the costs of a cleaning crew for both the house and the yard. After all the physical and emotional work that goes with planning, packing, and moving, most won't have an ounce of energy left for cleaning.
- There will always be some items that simply won't fit. Consider taking photos of those items and putting them in a book or see if the elder is ready to give away some of those treasures to loved ones.

What about the Beloved Pet?

One of the most painful challenges in planning a move may be making a decision about what happens to a loved pet. Discussing this issue in advance could allow time to find an apartment or assisted care facility that allows pets. According to federal housing laws, publicly run facilities cannot prohibit pet ownership as long as the elder is capable of caring for the pet. However, many private facilities and adult care homes do not allow pets. In that case, perhaps a family member or friend might be willing to keep the pet and bring the pet for visits. Some people, however, do not have friends or family willing to take on the responsibility. That leaves looking for a new owner.

While loved ones may advertise and interview perspective pet owners, often it is best to leave the process to professionals at "no kill" shelters. If friends and relatives do take on the task of finding a new home for the pet, they might first check with the veterinarian who has cared for the pet, the groomer, and other friends of the elder who may know of someone interested in taking in Fido or Chloe.

Once the pet is placed, ask the new owner to occasionally send notes and photos of the pet to help the elder feel confident the pet is being loved and enjoyed.

TWENTY TIPS TO HELP YOU GET RID OF JUNK

By Paula Spencer Scott for Caring.com
from https://www.caring.com/articles/getting-rid-of-seniors-junk
Reprinted by permission of Caring.com

Helping a parent downsize for a move can be complicated. Where you see a houseful of stuff to sort and toss, your parent is apt to see treasures, essentials, and a lifetime of memories. "To let go of what we have around us is to confront a very different living situation," says senior relocation industry leader Nan Hayes of Hinsdale, Illinois, founder of MoveSeniors.com. "People tend to cling to their possessions to avoid dealing with other issues, like stress or fear."

For adults over sixty, only a spouse's death and divorce rank as more stressful than moving to a nursing or retirement home, according to the Social Readjustment Rating Scale, aka the Stress Scale. Here are twenty expert-tested ideas to avoid the "junk wars" and make downsizing less stressful—for all of you.

How to Sort

1. **Avoid tackling the whole house in one go.** Though it's more efficient for you to plow full steam ahead, your parent is apt to be stressed emotionally, if not also physically. When organizing a parent's move, it's better to think in terms of months, not days. Tackle one room or area at a time. About two hours at a stretch is ideal for many older adults, says Margit Novack, president of Moving Solutions in Philadelphia and founding president of the National Association of Senior Move Managers.
2. **Frame decisions as yes-no questions.** Open-ended choices put a reluctant mover on the spot, raising stress. Avoid asking, "Which pots and pans do you want to keep?" Winnow them down yourself first, then present a more manageable yes-no option: "I've got your best frying pan, a large pot, and a small sauce pot. Does that sound good?" "Couching questions for yes-no answers provides the opportunity for the parent to feel successful so you can move on to the next thing," Novack says.

   Items that exist in abundance work especially well to presort: clothing, kitchenware, tools, and anything else you know the person has way more of than he or she will have space for.

3. **Use the new space as a guide.** Measure exactly how much closet or cabinet space the new place has (assisted-living communities will provide this information if you ask), and fill an equivalent amount of space as you sort. Mark off the comparable space so your parent has a visual guide.

   Beware of excessive multiples. In assisted living, your parent only needs one frying pan, one or two sets of sheets, one coffeemaker, one or two coats, and so on.

4. **Banish the "maybe" pile.** Relocation experts call it the OHIO rule: Only handle it once. The less decisive you are about what to do with an item, the more attached you (or your parent) risk becoming to it, Hayes says. Moving things in and out of "maybe" piles also takes time.

   As tempting as it is to set aside tough sorts for later, unless there's room to "hold" them at a relative's house, it's not generally worth paying storage-rental fees (unless it's a very large estate and time is tight). That's because once the items are boxed, your parent isn't likely to look at them ever again. (Out of sight, out of mind.)

   Exception: Save time by boxing piles of paperwork, which doesn't take much room. Papers are time-consuming to go through and present an unpleasant task for many disorganized people, casting a pall on your packing.

5. **Encourage your parent to focus on most-used items (and let the rest go).** Be patient and follow your parent's lead—what seems old and useless to you may be a source of great comfort and joy and therefore worth moving. "Don't go by the newest and best; go by what they use," Novack says. "You may think Mom should pack her pretty cut-glass tumblers for assisted living, but the reality is that those ugly, stained plastic ones are what she uses every day."

   When facing especially hard choices, ask for the story behind a dubious object—where it came from, when it was last used, whether a young family might put it to good use. This takes time, but the payoff is that, once your parent starts talking, he or she may have a clearer perspective and feel more able to let go, Novack says.

How to Cope with Treasures

6. **Pack representative bits of favored items (not the whole kit and kaboodle).** Photos, memorabilia, and collections typically take up far more space than the average assisted-living quarters can accommodate. Many services digitize images and papers for you for reasonable prices—sell the idea to your parent that every family member will get a copy, too. Pick key prints to display on the walls; large tabletop displays take up too much precious space.

7. **Cull a collection by asking, "Which is your favorite piece?"** Assure that one or two "best" items can have a highlighted location in the new home. "People sometimes feel OK about giving up the rest if they have a sense of control over the process," Novack says.
8. **Take photos of the rest of a collection and present them in a special book.** No, it's not exactly the same as owning, but it's a space-saving way for a collector to continue enjoying.
9. **If it's meant to be a gift or legacy, encourage giving it now.** Urge your parent not to wait for the next holiday, birthday, or other milestone to bestow; remind him that there's no space for storage. Ask, "Why not enjoy the feeling of giving right now?" (And if you're the recipient—just take it, and encourage your relatives to do the same. You can "lose" it later, if you don't want it, but the immediate need is to empty your parent's house.)

How to Sell

10. **Think twice before selling items on your own.** Craigslist, eBay, and other self-selling options are time-consuming when you're trying to process a houseful of goods. Be realistic: "The value of an item isn't what you paid for it or how well made or special it is. It's what someone is willing to pay for it," warns Novack.
11. **If there are several items of high value, consider an appraisal.** Go through the entire house; the appraiser will only come out once and is more interested in relatively large lots. Auction houses, whose goal is to sell items at the best price, are better options than antique dealers, whose goal is to get items for the lowest price, Novack says. Consignment shops will also sell items, but they tend to cherry-pick (they take fewer items) and often charge to pick up items.

How to Donate

12. **Understand how charities work.** The main donation outlets include Goodwill, the Salvation Army, AmVets, and Purple Heart. Depending on your area, popular alternatives may include other charities or a local hospital or PTA thrift shop. Senior living communities and moving companies often furnish lists of area charities that accept donations, says Nan Hayes of MoveSeniors.com. These charities work by selling castoffs; they don't want (and often won't take) dregs that are better left to the trash. Some take only furniture; some won't take clothing. Larger charities tend to accept a wider variety of items. Get a receipt for a tax deduction. Clarify whether they offer free pickup (a huge time-saver). Some charities will remove items from the ground floor only.

13. **Target recipients for specialty items.** It's time-consuming to find willing recipients for everything, but it may be worth the effort for items that your parent would be relieved to see in a good home. Examples: Schools may welcome musical instruments, old costumes, or tools. Auto repair shops and community maintenance departments may take tools and yard tools.

14. **Try the "free books" tactic.** In some communities, setting items on the curb with a sign that says "Free! Help yourself!" will make items miraculously disappear. This works great for books, Novack says, and sometimes other items. (Some libraries, charities, and schools take donated books and resell them, but finding a willing recipient and transporting the books—or any other items donated piecemeal—takes time.)

    In some areas, freecyling is an option. You post an item available for pickup to a membership list, and anyone who wants it can come pick it up from you (or from your curb). More than 5,000 groups make up the Freecycle Network (https://www.freecycle.org). Like selling items on Craigslist, however, the communications involved can be time-consuming and tedious if your goal is fast disposal of a large number of objects.

What to Discard

15. **If it's chipped, broken, or stained, toss it.** Charities don't want nonworking Christmas lights, snagged clothes, lidless plastic Tupperware, or any items that they can't sell. Period.

16. **Weigh your loyalty to recycling against your available time.** Avoiding waste is noble, but finding a home for every object can be incredibly time-consuming. "If you recycle the other 364 days of the year, tossing a few things in the interests of time is fine. You have to be pragmatic," Novack says.

17. **Don't be shy about tossing replaceable items without consultation.** Not worth moving, donating, or even conferring about: old spices, junk mail, old magazines (yes, even all those yellow-spined *National Geographic* issues), outdated medications, unused toiletries, plastic food containers, candles, stuffed toys (most charities won't accept them), and the contents of the junk drawer (just hang on to change and spare keys). Get rid of it when the homeowner isn't looking.

18. **For a price, you don't have to haul it away yourself.** The local garbage company may have limits on how many large black trash bags it will take, and not all local dumps take unsorted trash, either. Waste Management's Bagster (http://www.thebagster.com) is a smaller-scale alternative to a Dumpster, and it doesn't harm your driveway. Buy one of its large bags at a home-improvement retailer (about $30, depending on pickup location), fill with up to 3,300 pounds of trash, and call to schedule a pickup.

Services such as 1-800-Got-Junk (http://www.1800gotjunk.com/us_en) and 1-800-Junk-USA (which recently merged with the industry's other biggie, College Hunks Hauling Junk) (http://collegehunkshaul ingjunk.com) remove appliances and furniture as well as smaller items. Smaller local junk dealers may haul things away for free if they see, on appraisal, items that they'll be able to sell.

Get Help

19. **Consider bringing in the pros.** A fast-growing specialty, senior move managers specialize in helping older adults and are skilled at both the emotional and practical dimensions of late-life transitions. (The National Association for Senior Move Managers at http://www.nasmm.org has more than six hundred move-management company members.) These experts can defuse a parent-child emotional clash while handling everything from sorting and packing through hiring movers and unpacking in the new place. They usually charge an hourly fee that varies by locale.

20. **Investigate one-stop solutions if time is tight.** Deciding whether to sell, donate, give away, or throw away is stressful and takes a lot of time. Another way to outsource the tasks is to hold an estate sale. For example, Caring Transitions (http://caringtransitions.net) is a chain of senior-relocation franchises that handle estate sales.

Dealing with Downsizing Resources

AARP on "The Downsizing Dilemma": http://www.aarp.org/relationships/caregiving-resource-center/info-09-2010/ho_the_downsizing_dilemma.html

AARP on "How to Downsize Parents Who Might Be Hoarding": Online chat with moving and downsizing professionals answering questions about how to handle hoarding; http://blog.aarp.org/2011/10/10/caregiving-and-downsizing-your-parents-who-might-be-hoarder/

Aging Life Care Managers (ALCMs): http://www.aginglifecare.org

Downsizing and De-cluttering: http://states.aarp.org/downsizing-and-declut tering-kick-clutter-to-the-curb-sc-tn-wp-health/

Moving Elderly Parents: http://www.aplaceformom.com/senior-care-resources/articles/moving-elderly-parents

National Association for Senior Move Managers (NASMM) (http://www.nasmm.org): Can help you sort through the issues of transition and find professionals (senior move managers) in your area to help you move and/or downsize. For example, two Oregon companies that specialize in downsizing and moving elders are **Soft Landings for Seniors** http://www.softlandings forseniors.com and **Move-In Comfort** http://www.moveincomfort.com.

National Public Radio (NPR): Story on "Consultants Help Elderly Downsize at Home"; http://www.npr.org/templates/story/story.php?storyId=6460629

Pet Separation: http://www.aplaceformom.com/senior-care-resources/articles/ pet-separation

---

There's an App for That!

List Stuff Fast: Complete a photo inventory of your home with this app. https://itunes.apple.com/us/app/liststufffast-home-inventory/id922397384? ls=1&mt=8

Moving List: Get organized for your move with this iTunes app. https://itunes.apple.com/us/app/moving-list/id316092879?mt=8

My Move: Find a professional mover with this app. http://www.mymovingreviews.com/mobile-apps.php

---

For a downloadable form to keep track of **"My Move Mavens,"** go to https:// rowman.com/ISBN/9781442265462.

PROTECTING YOUR ELDER

EMERGENCY PREPAREDNESS

People of all ages should prepare for emergencies. Unfortunately, most of us don't take the necessary steps to create a plan and have the necessary supplies on hand. Here's a quick checklist to help you prepare for an earthquake, fire, hurricane, or other natural disaster. Also check out the links provided in this section for more detailed checklists of what to include in an emergency kit.

• **Create emergency kits.** Include the basics for first aid but also food and water supplies, blankets, flashlights and spare batteries, emergency hand-crank radio, candles, matches, paper, and pens. For a full list, see the link provided for the American Red Cross. The kits should be equipped for sheltering two weeks in place.

- **Have a spare battery or emergency portable charger for your cell phone.** These are small and fit in your purse or pocket.
- **Have a plan for where you will go for safety** in the event of each different type of disaster: hurricane, tornado, earthquake, fire, and flood.
- **Know all evacuation routes** in case your main road isn't accessible.
- **Have portable fire ladders** or "quick escape ladders" in every upstairs bedroom.
- **Share emergency plans** with others so they will know where and how to reach you.
- **Know where the water valve to your house is located.** If you are unable to turn it off, perhaps a neighbor can help, but you should know where to find the shut-off valve.
- **Similarly, know where your electrical power panel is** so that you can throw breakers in the event of a blackout.
- **Consider buying a generator** for backup power.

Emergency Resources

American Red Cross: Offers checklists of what goes in emergency kits, sells preassembled emergency kits, and offers emergency preparedness and first aid classes; http://www.redcross.org/prepare/location/home-family/get-kit

Center for Disease Control (CDC): Lists different types of emergencies and tips for preparing and safety; http://www.bt.cdc.gov/disasters/index.asp

Emergency Preparedness: http://www.ready.gov/

Federal Emergency Management Agency (FEMA): Features information on all types of emergencies and provides tips and booklets you can download; https://www.fema.gov/what-mitigation/plan-prepare

---

There's an App for That!

Go to your app provider and search for apps from **Red Cross**, **FEMA**, **HurricaneSoftware.com**, **Pocket First Aid and CPR**, **Ice Standard**, or **Disaster Alert**.

Specifically on Fire Prevention and Safety

After age sixty-five, people are twice as likely as the general population to be killed or injured in a fire. Making sure your elders have working fire detectors and fire extinguishers would be wise. Plus, here are some additional resources with ideas about fire prevention and safety:

Federal Emergency Management Agency (FEMA): Download free materials to train for fire safety; http://www.usfa.fema.gov/prevention/outreach/older_adults.html
National Fire Protection Association: Fire safety tips for seniors; http://www.nfpa.org/safety-information/for-consumers/populations/older-adults

PROTECTION FROM SCAMS

Everyone is at risk from scamming—on the Internet, by phone, through the mail, at your front door, on the bus, in the store. But elders are at a higher risk. Studies note that there are some common traits among elders that make them targets for scammers:

• Elders often don't pick up on warning signs such as a "smile on the face that doesn't extend to the eyes."
• They often are biased against negativity.
• They may live with day-to-day loneliness that leads to a willingness to listen to sales pitches.
• They have a natural desire to help.

Scammers are often very charming and caring and appear concerned for the elder's wellbeing. If visiting in person, a scammer may offer to fix something at no cost, or bring in the mail or a newspaper to gain the elder's trust. An elder may be suffering memory loss or dementia and, therefore, are unable to see through the scam. The elder may simply want to be helpful to another person. And elders may respond to scams because they are concerned about finances: If offered an "amazing deal to double his investment savings," an elder feeling financially insecure may jump at the opportunity. Sad but true, the scam may come from other family members or friends, so the elder may not suspect fraud.

Check out the detailed section on scamming in our "Financial" section. The following resources also offer the inside story on scams and how to avoid them.

AARP Quiz on "Are you an easy target for scammers?": http://www.aarp.org/money/scams-fraud/info-2014/scam-easy-target-quiz.html
Avoiding Credit Scams, Fraud, and ID Theft: http://www.aarp.org/money/scams-fraud/
National Adult Protective Services Association (APS): Find contact information for your state APS to report any type of adult abuse including scams; http://www.napsa-now.org/get-help/help-in-your-area/oregon/
National Council on Aging (NCOA): "Top 8 Ways to Protect Yourself from Scams"; http://www.ncoa.org/enhance-economic-security/economic-security-Initiative/savvy-saving-seniors/top-8-ways-to-protect.html

NCOA: "Top 10 Scams Targeting Seniors"; http://www.ncoa.org/enhance-economic-security/economic-security-Initiative/savvy-saving-seniors/top-10-scams-targeting.html

NCOA: "22 Tips for Avoiding Scams"; http://www.ncoa.org/enhance-eco nomic-security/economic-security-Initiative/savvy-saving-seniors/22-tips-for-avoiding-scams.html

HOUSING AND CARE PROVIDER CONCERNS FOR LESBIAN, GAY, BISEXUAL, AND TRANSGENDER ELDERS

Whereas the information we offer in *Eldercare 101* should apply equally regardless of race, color, religion, and gender, sadly, prejudice exists. If your elder is of a *racial* or *religious* minority, acceptance may be limited, but he is likely to find several available facilities and resources. Unfortunately, there is much less support for the LGBT community.

According to research, nearly three million elders age fifty-five and older in the United States identify as LGBT, and that number will double in the next two decades. LGBT elders are less likely to have children to support them in older years or to have someone help them plan or research their retirement options. Also, many are fearful about discrimination when it comes to assisted-care housing and in-home care.

Thanks to many LGBT-focused organizations, our society is experiencing a growing awareness of the challenges faced by LGBT elders who must deal with insensitive care providers. This awareness will lead to changes including LGBT sensitivity training and the hiring of LGBT care providers at mainstream facilities; the development of virtual retirement communities that value diversity; and the development of dedicated LGBT retirement communities such as the Fountaingrove Lodge. Check out the links for more information and, in particular, the Fountaingrove Lodge story from the *New York Times*.

More Information

"Aging Shows No Discrimination: Gay Seniors Search for Welcoming Assisted Living": Informative blog post; http://www.aplaceformom.com/blog/aging-shows-no-discrimination-gay-seniors-search-for-welcoming-assisted-living/

Assisted-Living Directory for LGBT-Friendly Facilities: http://www.assisted-living-directory.com/content/gay-friendly-facilities.cfm

"Graying and Gay, and Finding a Home": Article on Fountaingrove Lodge in Santa Rosa from *New York Times*; http://www.nytimes.com/2012/02/24/us/at-fountaingrove-lodge-in-santa-rosa-a-gay-retirement-community.html

A Look at Housing for Older LGBT Adults: Article on LGBT elder housing options; https://www.caring.com/articles/lgbt-senior-housing-options

National Resource Center on LGBT Aging: The country's first and only technical assistance resource center aimed at improving the quality of services and support offered to LGBT older adults; http://www.lgbtaging-center.org

"Out and Visible: The Experiences and Attitudes of LGBT Older Adults, Ages 45–75": Study exploring the aging realities of LGBT people as well as their fears, beliefs, behaviors, and aspirations in areas such as health care, finance and retirement, support systems, housing, and sources of information; http://www.lgbtagingcenter.org/resources/resource.cfm?r=695

FOR IMMEDIATE HELP TO DEAL WITH ABUSE
If a situation is serious, threatening, or dangerous,
call 911 or your local police for immediate help.
Or contact the Eldercare Locator on weekdays
for state specific information
at 1-800-677-1116.

ADULT PROTECTIVE SERVICES AND REPORTING ABUSE

Most of us have heard of elder abuse either through news stories, or perhaps you know of friends and neighbors who have been victims of abuse. It's shocking to think that anyone would prey on those who are most vulnerable and who often must depend upon others for some level of care. Often the abusers are well known to the elder; they might be family members or "friends."

According to the U.S. Government Administration for Community Living (ACL), "Elder abuse is a term referring to any knowing, intentional, or negligent act by a caregiver or any other person that causes harm or a serious risk of harm to a vulnerable adult." The ACL identifies primary types of abuse as: physical abuse, sexual abuse, neglect, exploitation, emotional abuse, abandonment, and self-neglect.

If you are a victim of abuse or suspect an elder is being abused and is in imminent danger, call 911. To report concerns about a caregiver or abuse that may be happening, contact the National Center on Elder Abuse to find a local agency; the link is provided at the end of this section.

One of the most active programs fighting abuse within care facilities is the federally mandated Long-Term Care Ombudsman Program. Every state must have an ombudsman program. Ombudsmen share information about complaints filed about care facilities and how those complaints were resolved. They also will respond to any calls about elder abuse and perform unannounced audits of facilities. If you suspect abuse of any type in a care facility, call your ombudsman immediately.

Need Help ASAP?

U.S. Department of Health and Human Services, Administration for Community Living (ACL) on "What Is Elder Abuse and What Are the Warning Signs?": http://www.aoa.gov/AoA_programs/elder_rights/EA_prevention/whatisEA.aspx

Find an Ombudsman in Your Area: http://theconsumervoice.org/get_help

National Adult Protective Services Association (APS): Where you can find contact information for your state APS to report any type of adult abuse; http://www.napsa-now.org/get-help/help-in-your-area/oregon/

National Center on Elder Abuse: http://www.ncea.aoa.gov/

Residents' Rights: http://www.ltcombudsman.org/about-ombudsmen#Residents_Rights

What Does an Ombudsman Do? http://www.ltcombudsman.org/about/about-ombudsman

MEDICAL PILLAR OF AGING WELLBEING

Make a habit of two things: to help; or at least to do no harm.

—Hippocrates

Chapter Five

Presto! You Have Thirty-five Extra Years to Live! Should You Spend Them Going from One Medical Appointment to Another?

Naturally, we are doing a happy dance when we consider all the wonderful gifts that have come with the extension of our lives thanks to scientific breakthroughs. Consider the incredible benefits of clean water and sanitation, antibiotics, and the developmental understanding about nutrition! With our additional years, we may have time to enjoy multiple careers, watch grandchildren grow up, mentor others, travel, experience deeper and longer-lasting relationships, and impact the world with our expanded wisdom.

However, despite this gift of longevity, our end-of-life years are inadvertently filled with chronic illness and suffering. The hope of all gerontologists is to see these years intentionally sprinkled back into the life course where they can be lived and enjoyed, after which we then compress illness toward the very end of life, closer to the period of time before we die. This gerontology dream will take intentional effort on the part of society. It must start at the childhood developmental stage. And we must integrate knowledge and health habits we know manifest good and long-lasting health into our lives *throughout* our lives.

There is no secret to healthy aging. We know what it takes. Research has proven time and time again that how we start out in the world directly impacts our aging trajectory. Poor access to health care and good nutrition as children directly correlates to the maladies of our older selves. If we look at the choice of investing what looks like small money on the front end of our lives when compared to the catastrophic expense we are paying for elder care and health care toward the end of our lives, there is no room for debate on the course we must take in America and in our own homes.

British chef Jamie Oliver is one of my favorite examples of a disrupter to the status quo. He tirelessly works to bring healthy food knowledge into our schools here in America. We can start aggressively by cutting out sugar and processed foods in our own homes. Often, the unhealthy choices are cheapest on the grocer's shelves. In response, we can create affordable healthy alternatives by starting a garden in a planter box or yard, joining a food co-op, teaching kids to cook, and so much more. This is an area where kids and elders can thrive together and expand the health of society. Of course, these are complex issues with many tendrils into our society, but we will not get there unless we put one foot in front of the other by starting with ourselves and those for whom we care.

A dear elder for whom I navigated care lived a very full and active life until her death at the young age of eighty-three. Georgina was tenacious with her drive for doing charity work and celebrating every day with family gatherings and healthy food. She was a dedicated grandmother, and she never missed an opportunity to try something new. She also had been very active with sports in her youth and looked after herself as she aged.

One day, her daughter called me to say she was seeing some unusual changes in her mother's behavior. She and her siblings assumed it was dementia and made arrangements with her doctor to test their mother's health. They had some health insurance issues to work through, so her appointments were delayed. As the days progressed, it became clear that Georgina was not able to be on her own. She became frustrated and depressed as she struggled to understand what was going on with her mind. I explained to the daughter that dementia causes a decline over time and that the changes presented by her mother seemed very sudden. I mentioned it sounded like a possible brain tumor or stroke and there was a real urgency to her being tested. That same week, the doctors discovered she did, in fact, have an inoperable brain tumor and hospice was started immediately.

Although hearing the diagnosis of their mother's condition was difficult, the family was empowered to step into planning mode for what time was left. The question of how long Georgina would suffer with dementia was no longer a mystery. She survived another month and died surrounded by her children and grandchildren. She lived her life fully until the end and then passed within six months of becoming ill.

Although saying good-bye is never easy, the suffering for Georgina and her family was compressed, while allowing her a fully engaged life until the end. She had time to be embraced by her family and then return to the stars.

As an ALCM, I know firsthand the hidden issues and resources needed for a successful medical navigation. For the "Medical" section of *Eldercare 101*,

I have asked Joyce Sjoberg and Dr. Ben Hellickson to address my specific concerns and pull together all the information needed to manage the medical maze during eldercare. Joyce is a registered nurse and certified ALCM, and Dr. Hellickson is a dentist who enjoys his elder patients. Throughout the section, Joyce shares how to choose your aging life medical care team as well as how to manage your elder's health records, medications, and therapy options. She also walks us through the process of aging with strategies and resources for healthy living and brings clarity to what brain disease really means. Dr. Hellickson helps us to understand the aging mouth and how our dental health affects our whole body.

Navigating the Medical Maze

Joyce Sjoberg, MA, RN, BSN, CMC

As your elders age, at some point, they will likely experience health-related problems, whether physical or mental. It's a fact: If we live long enough, our bodies eventually start to wear out, or some malady or another becomes a constant concern. As health deteriorates, the medical system takes center stage in an elder's life. Doctors' appointments, visits by occupational therapists, trips to the pharmacy—medical-centric activities—start to take up more and more time. Some elders get to know their medical support team so well they feel like family and even exchange holiday gifts!

In this section of *Eldercare 101*, we focus on the medical pillar of aging wellbeing, and we begin with prevention, the most important aspect of medical care. Then we cover everything you need to know about doctors and other medical support professionals. We highly recommend you help your elder(s) to build a healthcare medical "team," with a trusted primary care provider (PCP) as the team "captain." Having a geriatric specialist as the PCP after the age of sixty-five is optimum but not essential if the PCP has training in geriatrics.

After talking about the healthcare team in general, we delve deeper into the importance of dental and oral care in the lives of elders, explore the ins and outs of medical insurance, discuss the potential progressive stages of medical support, suggest ways to navigate the world of mental illness and brain disease, and, finally, review what to expect at the end of your loved one's life.

Before you delve into the "Medical" section, however, we challenge you to take the time to be sure you know where your elder keeps her Medicare or Medicaid cards and the names and phone numbers of her doctors and other healthcare team members.

To have a ready reference for getting in touch with these team members, we recommend you go to https://rowman.com/ISBN/9781442265462 and download the **"Medical Aging Life Care Team"** form.

We also would like to call attention to four particular documents that are of utmost importance when it comes to caring for our elders:

1. **Physician Orders for Life-Sustaining Treatment (POLST)**
2. **Advance Care Directive (also called Healthcare Directive or Advance Directive)**

3. **Healthcare Power of Attorney (HCPOA)**
4. **Health Insurance Portability and Accountability Act (HIPAA) Release**

These were addressed in the "Legal" and "Financial" sections, and they are so important that we repeat them over and over. These first two forms empower elders to outline their desires and wishes in advance of experiencing an emergency. They also allow you, caregivers, and medical personnel to adhere to those wishes when serious or life-threatening medical issues arise. The last two forms give designated individuals permission to speak with medical staff about their elder so they can assist with medical issues and paperwork. Communication is key when it comes to health care!

AN OUNCE OF PREVENTION

According to Benjamin Franklin, "An ounce of prevention is worth a pound of cure." The quote could be no more *apropos* than in relation to human health! We know that eating lots of green leafy vegetables can help prevent heart disease, that stretching or doing yoga daily can help keep our joints limber, and that learning a foreign language is good for our brains. In addition to eating well and exercising our bodies and minds, we also need regular checkups (medical and dental), deep, connecting social interaction, and getting outdoors to play!

When it comes to elders, staying on top of wellness activities is especially important. The longer someone stays healthy the better, partly because bouncing back from an illness or an injury when you're older can be an extra challenge.

In exploring wellness for elders, one of the places to begin is with general safety. Is your elder's living situation as accident-proofed as it can be for someone whose eyesight and balance is not what it used to be? Is there anything you can do to make her home safer? You will find the answers to these questions and more about safety in the "Living Environment" section of *Eldercare 101*.

Another extremely important component to wellness is having strong, fulfilling relationships. So critical to wellness are good quality relationships that we have devoted an entire section to social issues related to elders. In essence, it's good to remember that, although entertaining in their home, apartment, or even room can become overwhelming for your elders, they don't have to give up their friends. You can help them arrange theater or music dates; they might continue to attend worship activities or sing in a choir; another option is inviting friends to potlucks for which the guests all bring something and clean up, too. There are lots of activities elders can do with their friends that are comfortable and easy.

In this first section of our "Medical" chapter, however, we go beyond general safety. We begin our discussion with information on deterrents to wellness, in an effort to educate and advocate for making healthy choices. Then, in the rest of the section, we explore maintaining wellness through several research-proven elixirs for health.

DETERRENTS TO WELLNESS

Lack of Purpose

Getting older isn't easy. Changes in vision, hearing, dexterity, or mobility might make the activities we've enjoyed challenging and sometimes impossible. We might not be able to drive to attend events that would be emotionally, intellectually, or spiritually stimulating. Our children might have moved away, our partner might have died, and we might feel as though our world has gotten very, very small—and that our life has no purpose. Those who provide care for older adults must be vigilant to watch for signs that their elder has lost a sense of purpose. Some typical catch phrases of elders with this dilemma are: "Life doesn't matter" and "Don't worry about me."

If you fear your elder lacks a sense of purpose, help her find ways to reflect upon her significance in the lives of others. Facilitate her getting involved with activities she once enjoyed. Also, intergenerational activities can be a balm for lack of purpose, as can gardening, art, and music. The "Social" section of this book highlighted other options for nurturing wellbeing, which ultimately impacts sense of purpose.

Stress

By definition, *stress* is a state of mental or emotional strain or tension resulting from adverse or demanding circumstances. Mental or emotional stress results in physical reactions such as rapid heartbeat, frequent contraction and dilation of blood vessels, digestive problems, and overworked glands. One would think that after we retire our life would finally be stress free, as we no longer have the stressors that come from our work lives and caring for families. As we age, however, stress still complicates our lives! Finding ways to develop and create a lifestyle that includes a relaxed pace, slower rhythms, and less commitments is the first step to coping with stress at any age. Some tips include:

- Smile and laugh often.
- Think positive thoughts. You can't change situations, but you can change the way you think about and respond to particular events or situations.
- Get into nature often and breathe deeply.

- Practice an exercise that reduces stress and anxiety such as Tai Chi or Yoga.
- Explore and engage in mindfulness practices. Authors to explore on this topic include Donald Altman, Pema Chodron, Deepak Chopra, Jon Kabat-Zinn, and Thich Nhat Hanh—to name a few. Also, many videos, TED talks, and apps can be found online by searching for terms such as "stress reduction," "mindfulness," or "meditation."

Depression

Only 10 percent of older adults over the age of sixty-five are treated for clinical depression.[1] Does that mean that our elders just don't get depressed? No. Depression is often overlooked or misdiagnosed in elders either as situational grief, as a side effect of medications, or as a symptom of a disease. Well-meaning family members and friends also often mistake clinical depression in their elder for boredom or loneliness. They are all very different beasts! According to the National Institute of Mental Health, these are a few of the signs and symptoms of clinical depression:[2]

- Difficulty concentrating, remembering details, and making decisions
- Fatigue and decreased energy
- Feelings of guilt, worthlessness, and helplessness
- Insomnia, inability to sleep, waking up and feeling exhausted
- Feelings of hopelessness and pessimism
- Loss of interest in activities that brought pleasure in the past, including sex
- Overeating, undereating, or a significant loss of appetite
- Persistent pain, body discomfort, or symptoms that aren't relieved by usual treatment
- Ongoing feelings of sadness, anxiety, or an empty feeling
- Thoughts of suicide and talking about this to family or friends

If you suspect your elder is suffering from depression, reach out to her healthcare team and request that she be assessed. If the symptoms tend more toward boredom and loneliness, refer to our "Social" section to learn ways to promote social interaction.

Grief

Grief is the natural reaction to loss and change. The most common and best-understood trigger for grief is the loss of a spouse. If the spouse was receiving hospice services, the hospice team will provide ongoing grief support for the surviving spouse throughout the following year. This grief support can range from infrequent communication in the form of notes, letters, and phone calls to more frequent support groups or one-on-one counseling.

Grief, however, can come from a variety of other sources as well:

* Loss of a home
* Moving into a care facility
* Moving away from friends and community
* Inability to attend church and interact with a spiritual community
* Loss of a pet
* Loss of a friend

Various community and senior centers offer grief support and counseling, as do some professional organizations such as the Alzheimer's Association and National Parkinson's Foundation. Your elder's PCP also may offer specific suggestions, or ask your ALCM for area resources for grief counseling.

Poor Nutrition

Older adults who are unable or unwilling to make healthy food and nutritional choices are often at risk for problems in concentration, low energy, and an inability to make decisions or exercise sound judgment. Over time, choices in poor nutrition can result in weight loss or a lack of nutrients needed for health, healing, and disease management.

Lack of Exercise

Elders who are unable or unwilling to exercise for even short periods each day are at risk for both physical injuries and poorly functioning mental and emotional health.

Sleep Deprivation

Elders still need seven to eight hours of sleep per night.[3] Although many elders nap during the day, this still doesn't change how night sleep is an essential component of overall health and wellness. Lack of sleep or sleep disturbances in older adults is now thought to contribute to a variety of physical or mental illnesses such as stroke, mild cognitive impairment, diabetes, and heart disease, to name just a few.[4] If you are concerned about the quality or quantity of sleep your elder is getting, be sure to raise the issue with your elder's PCP.

Poor Social Network

We are learning, especially through studies such as the 90+ Study from the University of California at Irvine (UCI), about the importance of a strong social network. The 90+ Study, for example, shows that having a good social network can result in well-functioning mental capacity.[5] On the contrary, a lack of a social network can place your older adult at risk for physical injury and cognitive impairment.

Substance Abuse/Addiction

Similar to clinical depression, alcoholism and drug abuse in older adults is underdiagnosed and often hidden in many families. Reports show that some 17 percent of older adults over the age of sixty are either alcoholic or abuse prescription drugs[6]—and the problem isn't going away soon.[7] Many factors contribute to this high incidence of alcoholism and substance abuse among elders:

• Elders often have dwindling social support systems and may turn to drugs and alcohol to manage stressors.
• Many older adults don't have insurance benefits that provide access to drug treatment programs.
• Non-English-speaking minorities are further disadvantaged as the complexity of conversation required to diagnose substance abuse or addiction can result in misunderstandings during translation with interpreters.
• Many elders have trouble getting to their PCP or healthcare team appointments due to a lack of transportation and don't want to bother close family, friends, or neighbors.

If you suspect your elder suffers with substance abuse or addiction, speak to her PCP and ask for referrals to local or national treatment programs. You also might reach out to case managers through insurance companies to inquire about treatment programs and coverage. In addition, local mental health clinics or practitioners will know local resources for older adults, or you can check out the website of the National Council on Alcoholism and Drug Dependence at https://ncadd.org.

HEALTHY EATING AND LIVING

We've all heard the old adage, "You are what you eat." Truly, nutrition has been proven to be the cornerstone of health. Our food provides the necessary energy to do what we want to do every single day.

What's the right food to eat for optimum health? The latest research generally states that we should eat foods "close to nature," foods without a lot of modification. Also, we should enjoy what we eat.

The Food Pyramid from the U.S. Department of Agriculture that has dominated the last forty years of food science is now called "Choose My Plate." We are encouraged to divide that plate in half; 50 percent should be fruits and vegetables, whereas the other 50 percent should comprise a mixture of protein and grains, with grains being a larger portion than protein. See http://www.Choosemyplate.gov for a visual representation of "the plate."

Other "diets" based on this guideline include:

- Mediterranean Diet
- Anti-Inflammatory Diet
- Dash Diet
- Mayo Clinic Diet

All these diets emphasize eating plant-based food high in fiber, low in protein, high in omega-3 fatty acids, and high in flavonoids. Also, they all tout eating lots of fruits and vegetables while limiting saturated fat, alcohol, and sodium.

Food and the 90+ Study

Since 2003, UCI has been studying the oldest members of our population, the largest growing age group in the United States. Called the 90s+ Study, UCI's research is one of the largest studies of this demographic in the world. Over the last decade, the 90s+ Study has uncovered certain key factors that have been shown to promote longevity. Interestingly, as noted on the study's website, people who were overweight in their seventies lived longer than normal or underweight people, and people who drank moderate amounts of alcohol or coffee lived longer than those who abstained.[8] Check out more about the study at http://www.mind.uci.edu/research/90plus-study.

What Does Your Elder's Plate Look Like?

Consider what foods your elder eats on a daily basis. What foods does she like? Are there particular foods that should be added to her diet? If you see any red flags, you might want to consult with a dietician.

Getting Enough Exercise (Physical and Mental)

What does your elder do during most of her day? If it's watching TV, consider that a red flag. Granted, keeping up with a complex plot of a TV show can be good for your brain, but those who watch TV more than two hours a night have greater incidences of diabetes and heart disease, according to the Harvard School of Public Health.

In fact, nearly all research has found the most important thing anyone can do to stay healthy and keep her brain functioning at its best is to exercise.[9]

It also keeps you stronger and helps with balance to prevent falls. Even a fifteen-minute walk three times per week can help. This is why one of the most important ways you can support your elder through the aging process is by encouraging her to establish an exercise routine—and stick to it.

She can start small and possibly work up to doing some form of exercise daily. Many local hospitals, community centers, as well as parks and recreation programs offer specific classes for elders. Some suggestions for low-impact exercise include walking, ballroom dancing, Tai Chi, swimming, yoga, Nia, and biking. Recumbent bikes, in particular, are great alternatives for elders as these easy-to-ride, low-to-the-ground bikes can easily be adapted for various physical limitations. Ideally, the weekly exercise routine would include diverse activities that include the following components: aerobic, stretching, strength, and balance.

If your elder is a company insurance group retiree or part of a Medicare Advantage or Medicare Supplement health plan, she may already have a SilverSneakers membership. This active adult wellness program is offered to many Medicare plans across the nation. To find out if your elder's health plan offers the **SilverSneakers Fitness** program, visit the organization's health plan locator at https://www.silversneakers.com.

Just as exercising the body is critical to physical health, exercising the mind is key to mental health. Playing bridge, reading, doing crossword puzzles, studying a new language, and other challenging mental "gymnastics" are being shown to be preventive of cognitive issues. There also are online activities available for low monthly or annual fees through programs such as **AARP Brain Fitness** (http://brain.aarp.org/) and **Lumosity** (http://www.lumosity.com/).

Tracking Devices

Tracking activity encourages daily commitment to physical and mental exercise. These systems are a combination of wearable technology (smartphone, smart watch, etc.) and apps for monitoring, receiving, and storing data provided. Devices such as **FitBit**, **Nike Fuelband**, and **Samsung Gear Fit** are among many others jumping on the trend to track activity, calories, and even sleep. Some of these products are or will move into a role of providing additional health information. For more providers, search online for "activity trackers" and "exercise trackers."

For a simple downloadable **"Daily Exercise Log"** form, go to https://rowman.com/ISBN/9781442265462.

FIFTY-ONE WAYS FOR ELDERS TO ENJOY NATURE

Being outside in nature can bring a calming sense of wellbeing. The nature experience can be as simple as sitting on a bench at the local park, as fun as going on a picnic, or as structured as participating in outings and walks offered by a local senior center. Too often, though, elders wind up inside their houses, apartments, or nursing home rooms bored, lonely, and feeling helpless. They often feel too afraid and trapped in their failing bodies to even go outside. But nature doesn't have to seem a different lifetime away.

If your elder is ambulatory, encourage her to continue all the outdoor activities she always has loved—but seek ways to adapt the activity to the new level of energy and ability. For example, you may need to build raised beds for your elder to garden with ease. If your elder always loved fishing, you or someone else may need to join him rather than letting him head out alone.

Another way for elders to stay active outdoors is to participate in the many programs offered at local senior centers and community centers. From stargazing to neighborhood walks, activities planned by trained professionals in the field of parks and recreation balance just the right amount of activity with rest.

Even if your elder is limited in mobility, nature can still be in her life. Green plants can be brought into your elder's home or room. Vegetables or flowers can be grown in patio pots. Birds, fish, dogs, and cats can be wonderful companions. Also, you can take your elder to the many handicap-accessible parks and gardens with a walker or a wheelchair. To find what venues in your area are handicap accessible, search online for "[your city/state] handicap-accessible parks" or "[your city/state] handicap-accessible gardens."

To assist you in getting your elder back to nature, we've provided here a list of some ideas:

1. Garden
2. Stroll through a park
3. Feed the birds
4. Visit a public garden
5. Drive along the beach
6. Walk to the library
7. Observe the moon
8. Plan a picnic
9. Go canoeing
10. Make sun iced tea
11. Play cards on the patio
12. Enjoy a sunset from the balcony
13. Open the windows
14. Read outside under a tree
15. Visit a botanical garden
16. Take a drive in the mountains
17. Eat lunch *al fresco*
18. Barbeque
19. Swing with the grandchildren
20. Stargaze
21. Go fishing
22. Take outdoor photographs
23. Visit a nearby aviary
24. Go to a Little League game in the neighborhood
25. Learn about native trees in the area

26. Watch a parade
27. Make a flower bouquet (to give away)
28. Do stretching exercises in the yard
29. Walk to the mailbox
30. Bird watch
31. Check out a nearby nature conservatory
32. Create planter pots on the patio
33. Enjoy a cup of coffee on the deck
34. Walk a block and say hello to a neighbor
35. Visit the zoo
36. Identify different constellations
37. Go berry picking
38. Walk the dog
39. Learn the names of local birds
40. Sing around a fire pit
41. Water the garden
42. Plant a window-ledge herb garden
43. Fill a bird feeder
44. Attend a night event put on by a local observatory
45. Plant a scent garden and enjoy the smells
46. Watch the sunrise
47. Tell stories around a campfire
48. Join a walking group
49. Sit on a dock and watch the boats go by
50. Take up dragon boat racing
51. Smell the roses

MAKING TIME FOR JOY

Most of us live our lives waiting for the "golden years." What makes them "golden"? Is it the number of years, the volume of time we've lived, or, as one wise elder said, "Taking time along the way to smell the flowers"? If we take the appropriate steps, the retirement years *can* be filled with joy. As mythologist, author, and educator Joseph Campbell so aptly wrote, "Find a place inside where there's joy, and the joy will burn out the pain."[10]

Thousands (maybe more!) of books have been written on how to find joy in life, at any age. One common theme among all the authors, psychologists, and philosophers is: Follow your passion. Elders need to remember this—or be reminded of it—because the retirement years can be a time to become immersed in all kinds of activities, hobbies, and passions. Consider this Goethe quote: "Talent is developed in retirement; character is formed in the rush of the world."[11]

Some elders will take advantage of the many opportunities offered throughout our communities such as classes at community colleges, senior or community centers, and churches or local businesses; organized self-enrichment travel; arts performances; and the list goes on. Other elders may need a nudge to explore whether music, woodworking, nature, or volunteering makes their heart sing. Still other elders may worry that they have to be good at something before getting involved with it; they grew up in a time when learning was for one sole purpose: to get a job. We know better today! We know exploration and learning can be fun, bring us joy, and enrich our lives—at every age.

If your elder has particular passions or hobbies, great! Empower her to keep participating in them. If your elder hasn't found "joy," encourage her to try something new. A good first step is getting involved in a structured class. Art, music, or movement therapists are also great resources. See our "Social" section for specific ideas and resources.

TIME FOR MEDICAL SUPPORT

Most of us will become ill when the delicate balance of wellness tips into the negative. Some warning signs that the older adult in your life is unable to maintain health and remain well include but aren't limited to:

- **Weight Loss:** Could be serious, may be related to lack of energy to prepare a meal, or may be due to medication changes.
- **Balance Issues:** May be due to joint pain or something more serious. Whatever the cause, balance issues put the older adult at a high risk for falls.
- **Behavioral Change:** May be due to a wide spectrum of causes—from dementia onset to a urinary tract infection. Some common indicators are Dad's dirty clothing, Mom wearing the same clothes daily, Grandpa not shaving, Granny not combing her hair, angry disposition, seclusion, and so on.
- **Environmental Changes in the Home:** Do you notice spoiled food in the refrigerator? Is the laundry piling up, has the stove been left on, or have you found pans that have been scorched? Are the police being called to the home frequently? Are bills not being paid? If you answer "yes" to any or a number of these questions, consider it a red flag and try to determine the cause of the changes.

As your elder begins to fail, medical care comes more and more into play. Dr. Atul Gawande says it best in *Being Mortal*: "Until that last backup system inside each of us fails, medical care can influence whether the path is steep and precipitate or more gradual, allowing longer preservation of the abilities that matter most in your life."[12]

To help you understand the possible medical picture for your elder, this section will cover various topics on health care such as how to find health-care providers, what medical issues to watch, and where to locate supportive resources.

"CAPTAIN" OF THE HEALTHCARE TEAM: THE PCP

As your elder ages, she may have a variety of ailments and be referred to a number of specialists for care. So "your left hand knows what your right hand is doing," choose a healthcare team captain, called the **primary care provider (PCP)**. In fact, most medical insurance companies require a designated PCP when signing up, and some even mandate referrals from a PCP before the insurance will pay to see a specialist.

Having one person overseeing the entire aging life medical team for your elder can be life-saving. More often than not, that professional can ensure your elder is not taking drugs on top of drugs whose interaction might cause adverse reactions. The PCP also could watch out to ensure that medication dosing is appropriate; too many elders continue to take dosages of drugs that were prescribed years (and pounds) earlier!

A PCP could be a medical doctor (MD), a doctor of osteopathy (DO), or a naturopathic doctor (ND). He or she also might be a nurse practitioner (NP) or a physician's assistant (PA).

Medical Doctor: An MD has attended and graduated from a conventional (allopathic) medical school. Within the MD option, you also have the choice of:
- **Family Practitioner:** Physician trained to provide care to an individual and all family members regardless of age, gender, or medical diagnosis.
- **Internist:** Physician who most often cares for adults and their medical needs. Patients usually range from older adolescents through older adults. Some internists continue to study an area of sub-specialty (neurology, orthopedics, pulmonology, etc.).
- **Geriatrician:** Internist or family physician specially trained in the care of older adults (generally defined as seventy-five years of age and older). This type of MD tends to focus on complex medical and social issues related to aging.
- **Hospitalist:** Specializes in hospital care and can coordinate and provide treatment in place of a PCP when the patient is hospitalized.

Doctor of Osteopathy: A DO is a fully trained and licensed doctor who has attended and graduated from a U.S. osteopathic medical school. The major difference between osteopathic (DO) and allopathic (MD) doctors is that some osteopathic doctors provide manual medicine therapies such as cranial-sacral work, spinal manipulation, or massage therapy, as part of their treatment, whereas MDs do not.

Naturopathic Doctor: NDs practice what is called naturopathy, a distinct system of primary health care that emphasizes prevention and the self-healing process through the use of natural therapies.

Nurse Practitioner: A NP is qualified to treat certain medical conditions without the direct supervision of a doctor. NPs diagnose and treat health conditions with an emphasis on disease prevention and health management.

Physician's Assistant: A PA is a highly trained, educated, and qualified medical professional who assists physicians and carries out routine clinical procedures under the supervision of physicians.

WHO'S THE RIGHT PCP FOR YOUR ELDER?

Having a geriatrician overseeing your elder's health care is ideal, but there currently is a shortage of geriatricians in the United States. Good family practitioners, internists, osteopaths, naturopaths, nurse practitioners, and physician's assistants can quite ably care for your elder.

If the current PCP is working well for your parent, great. If it's time to find someone new, make that happen. A good relationship with a PCP can be instrumental in preventing fear, frustration, disappointment, and anger during this stage of life that can be fraught with medical issues. The last thing anyone needs is not to trust and be able to count on the healthcare team "captain"!

When evaluating your elder's PCP or choosing a new one, consider the following points:

- **Your elder's expectation of the relationship:** Some people value long-term relationships and specifically look for a PCP who plans to maintain her practice for her entire career in the same area. Others value the ability to have immediate care—no matter who the doctor, nurse practitioner, or physician's assistant is—and prefer to be seen in retail clinics.
- **Service:** Consider how office staff members respond to your elder's calls, how they greet her while at the clinic, how responsive they are to urgent requests, and how they follow up on medical problems and agreements to assist your elder with ongoing care or referrals.
- **Communication:** Look for a PCP who discusses health and medical concerns in a way that meets your elder's needs. Does your elder prefer someone who gets directly to the point, someone who communicates as if you were a dear family member, or someone in the middle of the road?
- **Accessibility:** Can your elder reach her PCP directly or does she have to talk to the office staff first? Does it matter either way? Does the PCP offer direct e-mail contact, allowing you to reach her as concerns and questions arise? Are medical records accessible online through a secure medical records system?

- **His or her treatment approach:** Approaching the treatment of medical issues can take many forms. Some PCPs prefer to take a more conservative approach and recommend the treatment with the least impact to your life versus an aggressive approach with more impact. Keep in mind, the treatment with least impact can require considerably more effort on your part. PCPs also can vary in their focus: Some focus on treating medical issues, whereas others focus on wellness and prevention.
- **Team player:** Does your elder's PCP refer her to others who might offer different treatment approaches or a wellness plan?
- **Partner in health:** Does your elder believe her PCP strives to create a partnership with her and your family when it comes to making healthcare treatment decisions?

Plan a First-Time Visit with the New PCP

Before deciding on a new PCP, plan to meet and interview the PCP to determine if he is a good fit. Some PCPs will not charge for that first-time interview. Others might charge a "visit fee." Double check this in advance so your elder is not surprised if she gets a bill.

A SPECIALIST FOR THIS, SPECIALIST FOR THAT

Medical specialists are doctors who have completed advanced education and clinical training in a specific area of medicine. In addition to geriatricians and hospitalists (who can serve as PCPs), other examples of medical specialists (and their specialty areas) include:

Allergist (Immunologist): Immune system
Cardiologist: Heart
Dermatologist: Skin
Endocrinologist: Endocrine glands (regulate hormones)
Gastroenterologist: Digestive system
Geriatric psychiatrist (also known as **geropsychiatrist** or **geripsychiatrist**): Subspecialist of psychiatry who deals with the study, prevention, and treatment of mental disorders in elders
Hospice and Palliative Medicine Specialist: Prevents and relieves suffering of patients who have a serious illness or who have only a short time left to live
Infectious Disease Specialist: Complex or chronic infections
Nephrologist: Kidney and urinary system

Neurologist: Brain (such as dementia and Alzheimer's disease), spinal cord, and nervous system diseases or injuries

Oncologist: Cancer

Orthopedist: Bones

Ophthalmologist: Eyes

Pain Management Specialist: Specializes in treatment of people who have chronic pain, such as back pain or nerve pain from diabetes. Medical doctors from many different specialties such as anesthesiology, neurology, or physiatry might further specialize in pain management.

Pathologist: Examines tissue and blood samples to diagnose disease

Physiatrist: Specializes in helping people regain function after surgery, stroke, or injury

Podiatrist: Feet, ankles, and lower legs

Psychiatrist: Mental health problems such as depression

Pulmonologist: Lungs

Radiation Oncologist: Uses radiation therapy to treat people with cancer

Radiologist: Does imaging tests such as X-rays, ultrasounds, and MRIs; may also supervise people who perform tests such as barium enemas or CT scans

Rheumatologist: Joints

Sleep Disorders Specialist: Specializes in the diagnosis and surgical and nonsurgical treatment of sleep disorders such as sleep apnea and snoring

Surgeon: Evaluates people who have potential surgical problems and performs surgical operations and techniques; many subspecialties in surgery including chest (thoracic) surgery; blood vessel (vascular) surgery; mouth or jaw (oral/maxillofacial) surgery; and bone, muscle, and joint (orthopedic) surgery. Surgeons may further specialize by limiting their practice to specific age groups.

Urologist: Urinary system in men and women and disorders of the male reproductive system

Insurance Tip: Many medical insurance companies require a referral from a primary care provider before they will pay for the services of specialists.

DA FEET, DA FEET, DON'T FORGET DA FEET!

One specialist we listed in the last section who has an important but often overlooked role is the podiatrist, a doctor specializing in the foot, ankle, and lower leg. The reason the importance of the podiatrist is often overlooked is because feet are generally overlooked—until they become a problem! With routine care, some of the problems might be avoided. Also, some individuals with chronic illnesses such as diabetes are at higher risk for infections, skin breakdown, and other disease. For them, regular foot care is extremely important—like brushing teeth twice daily.

Some typical podiatry services include:

- A visual inspection of the feet, toenails, and skin up to mid-leg
- Treatment of and removal of dead skin pertaining to corns and callouses
- Cutting, clipping, trimming, or debriding toenails
- Recommendations for preventive maintenance care such as cleaning and soaking the feet and using skin creams to maintain skin tone
- Prescribing and fitting orthotics, insoles, casts, and custom-made shoes
- Ordering and performing physical therapy

Podiatrists usually have independent practices. If your elder is unable to leave home for podiatry services, you will want to find alternatives to visiting the podiatrist's office. Depending on where your elder lives, some podiatrists are now making home visits. Otherwise, home health nurses also can provide foot care. All registered, licensed practical, and licensed vocational nurses can legally care for feet and cut toenails under their scope of care.

Just as with any healthcare service, charges will vary depending on where your elder lives. Whereas some podiatry services for certain diseases are covered by most medical insurances, including Medicare and Medicaid, the reimbursement seems to be slow when it comes to home podiatry services. Because of this slow insurance processing for podiatry, it isn't unusual for healthcare professionals providing home podiatry and nail care services to ask for and receive reimbursement when services are rendered and then for the professional to reimburse the elder later, once the insurance company has paid her.

To find a podiatrist for your elder, start by asking his PCP for a referral.

SLP, PT, OT . . . OH, MY!

In addition to specialists who are doctors of medicine, other healthcare professionals are highly trained and certified to provide evaluative and hands-on therapies that help patients to improve their health and wellbeing. Most likely, the elder in your life will be referred by her physician to one or more of these specialists at some point during her aging process. It pays to know your elder's options.

Acupuncturist: Trained and certified individual who practices the originally Chinese wellness modality of inserting fine needles through the skin at specific points to cure disease or relieve pain. Acupuncturists also offer acupressure, which is applying pressure to the specific points of the body without inserting needles.

Art Therapist: Therapist who works to improve overall physical, emotional, and spiritual health through art and all its modalities (e.g., drawing, painting, or sculpture).

Audiologist: Person trained to evaluate hearing loss and related disorders including balance (vestibular) disorders and tinnitus (ringing in the ears) and to rehabilitate individuals with hearing loss and related disorders.

Breathwork Specialist: An umbrella term for various New Age practices in which the conscious control of breathing is meant to influence mental, emotional, and physical state—sometimes to claimed therapeutic effect.

Dietician: Trained and certified professional who advises people on what to eat in order to lead a healthy lifestyle or to achieve a specific health-related goal.

Feldenkrais Method Practitioner: This movement discipline aims to reduce pain or limitations in movement, to improve physical function, and to promote general wellbeing by increasing students' awareness of themselves and by expanding students' movement repertoire.

Horticultural Therapist: Therapist who works to improve overall physical, emotional, and spiritual health through the modalities of gardening, pruning, growing plants, flower arranging, and designing gardens.

Music Therapist: Therapist who works to improve overall physical, emotional, and spiritual health through the modality of music.

Occupational Therapist (OT): Highly trained professional who works with people to enhance their ability to engage in everyday activities. The OT does this by teaching new techniques to do everyday activities, providing equipment that facilitates independence, and recommending environmental (or home) modifications that support independence. Like PTs, OTs work in a variety of settings such as hospitals, nursing homes, private practices, outpatient clinics, and home health agencies.

Physical Therapist (PT): Highly educated, state-licensed healthcare professional who can help patients reduce pain and improve or restore mobility through exercises, manipulation, massage, and other modalities—in many cases without expensive surgery and often reducing the need for long-term use of prescription medications and their side effects. In addition, the PT works with individuals to prevent the loss of mobility before it occurs by developing fitness- and wellness-oriented programs for healthier and more active lifestyles. PTs work in a variety of settings as noted for OTs.

Speech-Language Pathologist (SLP) (also known as a Speech Therapist): Highly trained professional who identifies, assesses, and provides remediation for speech and communication disorders. The SLP's approach varies depending on the disorder and may include physical exercises to strengthen the muscles used in speech (oral-motor work), speech drills to improve clarity, or sound production practice to improve articulation.

Note: Most insurance companies will pay for the services of OTs, PTs, SLPs, and audiologists *with a doctor's referral*, but that is not the case with some of the other healthcare professionals. You need to read the fine print of your elder's insurance plan to verify coverage.

Resources for Finding Healthcare Providers

If your elder is new to an area or looking for a referral for healthcare providers, consider asking the following individuals or associations. Remember, however, despite someone else's opinion, your elder is often the best judge of who is the best fit for her.

- **Your parent's current (or past) PCP** (if available)
- **Family, friends, and neighbors**
- **Other specialists your elder already sees and trusts** (dentist, optometrist, ophthalmologist, pharmacist, etc.)
- **Local medical and/or disease specific associations** (search online for American Diabetes Association [plus state]," "American Cancer Society [plus state]," "Parkinson's Association [plus state]," etc.)
- **Local professional organizations** (search online for "American Medical Association [plus state]," "Aging Life Care Managers Association [plus state]," "Nurse Practitioners [plus state]," or "Physician's Assistants [plus state]")
- **Local area hospital or insurance groups** will have referral lines, although they are only able to share identifiable information (e.g., demographics, background and training, and specialty areas).
- **Insurance companies and/or Medigap programs** also have "find a healthcare practitioner" tools on their websites.
- **Local ALCMs** working in your community

There's an App for That!

http://www.betterdoctor.com: Find a new doctor, dentist, or other specialist.
http://www.doctorondemand.com: Have live video appointments with medical professionals.
http://eldercare.gov/Eldercare.NET/Public/Index.aspx: Find doctors, other healthcare practitioners, or health services in your area.

For a **"Potential Healthcare Providers"** form for collecting referrals, go to https://rowman.com/ISBN/9781442265462.

TIPS TO CONSIDER WHEN USING
A NEW HEALTHCARE PROVIDER

Insurance: Be sure to verify the provider will accept your elder's medical insurance plan.

Payment: Inquire about the health insurance documentation and the payment process required for receiving care. Note the contact information for the business administrator or the billing manager.

HIPAA: If you, as a caregiver, will be helping your elder with medical issues and paperwork, have your elder fill out the appropriate HIPAA release form to give you permission to speak with the medical staff. Do this before an emergency happens!

Office contact information: Be sure and ask if there is an office "team." For example, does the doctor have a back-line for a medical assistant you or your elder can call in an urgent situation?

Making appointments: What are the hours to call for appointments? Are there no-show policies? Can they provide estimates of waiting times, both for an appointment and when waiting to see the doctor after arrival?

After-hours and emergency care: Inquire about when to seek, who to call, and where to go for after-hours and emergency care.

Prescriptions: Obtain instructions for securing prescription refills, reporting adverse side effects, and decisions to discontinue medication or change any agreed-upon treatment plans.

Medical records: Ask about any instructions for bringing a summary of medical history, current health status, and recent test results, or if referral documentation is needed (especially important for specialists and testing).

Tests and test results: Request a description of what types of tests are commonly conducted in the practice and what tests are done by an external provider (with names and contact numbers for commonly used laboratories and radiology facilities). Find out the practice policy about patient notification of test results.

Special needs: Inquire if and how the provider can accommodate any unique or special needs (such as physical navigation, hearing or visual impairments, translation services, etc.), and how to arrange for assistance if needed.

Care companion: Notify the doctor's office if your elder plans to bring a companion or professional ALCM along with her to visits.

PREPARING FOR HEALTHCARE APPOINTMENTS

When we visit a doctor, we usually have three overall goals: (1) To communicate current needs and symptoms, (2) to understand the diagnosis, and (3) to discuss the treatment options. That's a lot to cover in the fifteen to twenty minutes that doctors usually schedule for appointments. This means we need to be as prepared as possible for the appointment and get all our questions asked and answered—leaving with a mutually agreeable treatment plan. Certainly, some appointments are urgent and can't be prepared for in advance, but, if we prepare for those appointments, we will be considerably more pleased with the outcome of medical office visits.

Here are a few suggestions of how your elder can prepare for a medical appointment:

1. **Write down her symptoms and anticipate the questions the doctor might ask.** She can use a smartphone to track symptoms, either by recording comments each day through audiotaping or by writing notes on a calendar.

> Another option is to fill out the **"Symptom Tracker"** form available at https://rowman.com/ISBN/9781442265462, or your elder's own version of it, to describe and track symptoms.

2. **Research the symptoms.** By doing prior research, your elder will better understand the possible causes of her symptoms and what the treatment options may be. Also, once she has a few ideas what might be occurring, she will be more prepared to discuss concerns with the medical provider and to understand the treatment recommendations.

   A number of options exist for where to do the research. One can start with the Internet and look for reputable online resources. (See our "Can I Trust the Internet for My Health Information?" page at the end of this section.) If you and your elder do not have access to the Internet nor know how to use a computer as an information resource, check out these places:

- **Nearest public library.** Ask to speak with a reference librarian. Reference librarians are trained to help find specific information.
- **Nearby hospital or healthcare system.** These institutions often have medical libraries, many of which are staffed with medical reference librarians who can help research specific symptoms, questions, and concerns.
- **Nearby local associations specific to the medical concerns**. These organizations are staffed with professionals trained to provide information and resources with a focus on their specific disease (e.g., American Diabetes Association, American Cancer Association, and Parkinson's Association).

3. **Write down three to five specific questions for the doctor.** Sample questions include:
   - How will this diagnosis or illness affect my day-to-day life?
   - Why do you recommend this test and are there any risks associated with it?
   - Are other treatments available? If so, when will we discuss those options?
   - How will this medicine help me and how soon can I expect it to work?
   - What are the possible side effects of this medication or treatment?
   - Where can I get more information and support for my illness?
   - How soon should I see you again so we can review test results and discuss my progress or options in greater detail?

4. **Plan ahead to bring along a trusted advisor.** This can be a family member, friend, or hired ALCM. The role of this advocate is essential in health care. When anyone is stressed, sometimes only 25 percent of what is being asked or said is heard and understood.

ON THE DAY OF A HEALTHCARE APPOINTMENT

Bring:
- Insurance cards
- Picture ID
- Symptom tracker form (or other written notes about symptoms)
- List of questions
- List of medications (both prescribed and over the counter)
- Diagnosis list
- Water and snacks (delays happen)
- Prepared "just-in-case" kit (including the likes of extra underwear, incontinence briefs, phone charger, towelettes, hand sanitizer, light blanket, small flashlight, etc.)

Call the provider's office thirty to sixty minutes before arriving to ensure the office is running on time. If not, you might consider waiting longer before leaving for the appointment. Some older adults do not have the attention span to wait and will begin to behave in ways that will detract from the reason for the appointment. Others might become too tired for the appointment.

Leave plenty of time (in fact, extra) to get to the appointment. If you're the caregiver, this includes arriving at your elder's home prepared she might not be ready (e.g., dressed, know where the keys are to lock up the home, and have gas in the tank if you need to take her car).

Keep in mind the goals for the particular office visit. Some possible examples are:

- Discuss new symptoms and get medical provider to diagnose and treat.
- Discuss recent changes and get support.
- Discuss urgent medical issues or concerns.
- Clarify next steps, possible referrals, and where to go next for the best medical care or treatment.

Tip: Remind your elder to keep focused on the goals and don't let herself get off track.

Ask questions any time something doesn't make sense. For example, you might not understand a word or terminology describing a medical test, medication or procedure, or a possible treatment option.

Be open and honest with the provider, even if the discussion feels uncomfortable. Without honesty, the medical provider ultimately can't help.

Be sure to ask the questions you came with. For example, are there other ways to treat this problem that don't involve all these medications? Or, to whom do we talk about the treatment and medication costs?

Request written materials about the diagnosis or follow-up treatment. These materials can be helpful to review at home.

Request a copy of the "after-visit note." These notes detail what was said in the visit, recommendations made, and any new medications and treatments.

CHECKLIST OF WHAT TO PACK FOR A HOSPITAL STAY

At some point, your elder may need to be hospitalized because of a fall, for a procedure, or in the event of a major health crisis. Whatever the reason, your elder doesn't need to bring much for the stay. In fact, she may want to have a bag packed, just in case, with the following items:

- Medication list
- Copies of POLST, advance directive, and HCPOA forms
- Robe and rubber-soled slippers (if she won't want to wear the rubber-soled socks the hospital usually gives to patients)
- Personal toiletries such as toothbrush, toothpaste, deodorant, razor, lip balm, and denture cream
- Watch, clock, and calendar
- Books, magazines, or crossword puzzles
- Small amount of cash (no more than $20) for vendors
- Snacks or protein nutritional supplements that aren't heat and time sensitive and can provide much-needed protein and calories when hospital cafeterias aren't open late at night
- Put in at the last minute: Eyeglasses, hearing aids, dentures, cane/walker, and cell phone and charger
- Only include if there's a safe storage place in the hospital room: iPad, Kindle, iPod, or other electronic device for entertainment
- **Leave home: Jewelry, wallet, and anything else of value**

HIGH-TECH MEDICATION SUPPORT

According to the National Center for Health Statistics, 40 percent of elders take five medications or more. Forty percent of the time, elders take their medications incorrectly by forgetting them, confusing their meds, or double dosing.[13] While the challenges of taking medications correctly cannot be fixed with technology, some medication dispensers and reminder apps can help. Although many apps are now available, here is a sampling:

Medication Dispenser Systems

ePill: http://www.epill.com/dispenser.html
Med Minder: http://www.medminder.com
Med Ready: http://www.medreadyinc.net/cart2/
Med-e-Lert: http://www.medelert.net/

Medication Reminder Apps

Med Coach: https://itunes.apple.com/us/app/medcoach-medication-reminder/
Drugs.com: http://www.drugs.com/apps/
One hundred apps for medication reminders: http://appcrawlr.com/ios-apps/best-apps-pill-reminder

Text Reminders

Med Texter: http://www.medtexter.com/

All the Above

GlowCap by Vitality: http://www.vitality.net
Twist-off cap blinks and chirps when it is time for a dosage, while a separate plug-in wall unit glows and emits escalating alerts for two hours. Then it dispatches e-mails and phone calls, including "buddy reminders" to family members or caregivers. You press a button beneath the cap to arrange for a refill.

For a simple, downloadable **"My Medications"** form, go to https://rowman.com/ISBN/9781442265462.

HOW TO DISPOSE OF OLD OR UNWANTED MEDS

Medications are important for a variety of medical and health reasons. When a medication is no longer ordered or needed, has been discontinued, or has expired, what happens to those unused pills or liquid? They must be disposed of properly to avoid being possibly ingested by anyone other than the person for whom the medicine was prescribed; even a single dose of some medicines can be lethal. Also, improperly disposing of drugs can be harmful to the environment and pets.

Because of the importance of properly disposing unwanted and expired meds, the U.S. Department of Justice's Drug Enforcement Administration offers city and county "take-back" programs. Contact your city or county government's household trash and recycling service to see if there is a medicine take-back program in your community and learn about any special rules regarding which medicines can be taken back. You also can talk to your pharmacist to see if she knows of other medicine disposal programs in your area, or visit the U.S. Drug Enforcement Administration's website for information on National Prescription Drug Take-Back Events at http://www.deadiversion.usdoj.gov/drug_disposal/takeback/.

Interestingly, some especially harmful medicines should be flushed down the sink or toilet if the medicine is no longer needed—to absolutely ensure that they will not be accidentally ingested by children, pets, or anybody else. Note that disposal by flushing is **not** recommended for the vast majority of medicines. For information on drugs that should be flushed, visit the FDA website at http://www.fda.gov/downloads/Drugs/ResourcesForYou/Consum ers/BuyingUsingMedicineSafely/EnsuringSafeUseofMedicine/SafeDisposal ofMedicines/UCM337803.pdf.

If you and your elder live in a location that is inconvenient for participating in drug take-back programs, then consider disposing of medications at home. To do so:

- Place the unwanted medication in a plastic bag that can be securely sealed or in a disposable container with a lid (such as a margarine tub).
- Mix the drug with an inert material such as used coffee grounds or kitty litter.
- Add a liquid such as soda, water, or an over-the-counter liquid medication no longer needed (such as an antacid medication).
- Seal the disposable container or plastic bag and throw in your household trash.
- Conceal with duct tape, cross out with black permanent marker, or scratch off any personal information, including the Rx number, on the empty medicine containers before throwing them into the trash.

For liquid medications, mix the liquid with an absorbent substance such as flour or kitty litter to help discourage misuse or unintentional use.

TO VACCINATE OR NOT TO VACCINATE?

The CDC estimates that one million Americans contract shingles every year. About half of these individuals are over the age of sixty. Additionally, more than 60 percent of seasonal flu-related hospitalizations occur in people sixty-five years and older.[14] The numbers are not surprising. As we age, our immune system tends to weaken, putting us at higher risk for certain diseases. This is why, in addition to the seasonal flu (influenza) vaccine and the Td or Tdap vaccine (tetanus, diphtheria, and pertussis), elders also should get:

- Pneumococcal vaccine, which protects against pneumococcal disease including infections in the lungs and bloodstream (recommended for all adults over sixty-five years old).
- Zoster vaccine, which protects against shingles (recommended for adults sixty years or older).

If your elder travels outside of North America or has other healthcare conditions, other vaccinations may be warranted. Be sure to discuss this topic with your elder's PCP.

For a form to track **"Keeping Up with Checkups and Vaccines,"** go to https://rowman.com/ISBN/9781442265462.

CAN I TRUST THE INTERNET FOR HEALTH INFORMATION?

Not all Internet sites are created equal! Here are five questions to ask yourself before you trust the health information you find online:

1. **Who runs this site?** For example, is the site run by a national organization versus an individual who has the medical condition you are exploring.
2. **Who is paying for this site?** Is the site advertising? If so, what is being sold? Does the information seem to favor particular products and services?
3. **Is the site run and written by experts?** Click on the "About Us" tab to see if experts are listed for the medical condition you are researching. Beware of sites offering personal "medical" opinion versus information stated by experts and supported by research.
4. **Is the site asking for my elder's personal information?** If so, be sure you know the site's privacy policy so you know how your elder's personal information will be shared.
5. **Is the site reviewed annually, at a minimum?** Does it contain up-to-date information?

Some Reputable Online Medical Resources

American College of Physicians (ACP): https://www.acponline.org/patients_families/products/health_tips/; ACP has an easy-to-understand tool called "HEALTH TiPS." This tool allows you to click on a particular disease or diagnosis and download and print out a free information sheet on the topic (in English or Spanish). The sheet also includes questions to ask during a PCP appointment, along with space to write the answers.

Healthfinder.gov: http://www.healthfinder.gov is managed by the U.S. Department of Health and Human Services; features a variety of health topics and general information.

Health in Aging: http://HealthinAging.org; Created by the American Geriatrics Society's Health in Aging Foundation by trusted professionals in the field of geriatrics. Provides consumers and caregivers with up-to-date information on health and aging.

Medline Plus: http://www.nlm.nih.gov/medlineplus/; A good one-stop shop for basic health information provided by the U.S. National Library of Medicine and National Institutes of Health. The site includes a medical encyclopedia to look up tricky words, information on hundreds of prescriptions by brand name, and links to doctors, hospitals, and medical libraries across the country.

National Health Information Center: http://www.health.gov/nhic; this website, part of the National Institutes for Health system, lists more than 1,400 organizations and government offices that can provide free health information upon request. Actually, for a quick online rundown on a condition, this might be the best place to start searching. This site allows you to search for information on a condition by its location in the body, by the disease name, or by health issues.

WebMD: http://www.webmd.com; a reliable standby in the online medical universe. The site offers much of the same general information as the government sites mentioned previously, but its style is extremely user-friendly and created with the general consumer in mind.

MEDICAL INSURANCE

This section is intended to help individuals and their family members understand what is and isn't covered by medical insurance. Knowing what isn't covered can help someone budget and make sometimes complex healthcare decisions later in life.

PAYING FOR AND/OR GETTING
REIMBURSED FOR MEDICAL CARE

As noted in our "Financial" section, our government as well as private pay companies offer health insurance. The primary medical and health insurance policies available for elders are:

1. **Medicare**
   • Medicare Part A (Hospital Insurance)
   • Medicare Part B (Medical Insurance)
2. **Private Pay Supplemental Health Insurance**
   • Medicare Advantage Plans (Medicare Part C)
       Health Maintenance Organization (HMO) Plans
       HMO Point-of-Service (HMOPOS) Plans
       Preferred Provider Organization (PPO) Plans
       Private Fee-for-Service (PFFS) Plans
       Special Needs Plans (SNPs)
       Medical Savings Account (MSA) Plans

Medicare Supplement (Medigap) Insurance
- Medicare Part D (Prescription Drug Coverage)

3. **Medicaid** (has strict asset and disability requirements)

Your elder also might have some medical and healthcare costs covered by:

- **LTC Insurance**
- **Veterans Affairs (VA) Aid & Attendance (A&A) Benefits**
- **Private Insurance**

In addition, some people use income from the following toward their medical expenses:

- **Social Security**
- **Supplemental Security Income (SSI)**
- **Special Needs Trusts**

Tip: Navigating the medical and health insurance maze of coverage and options can be a challenge. An ALCM can help guide you and your elder through it.

WHAT MEDICARE COVERS

Medicare[15]—the red, white, and blue paper ID card—is the federal health insurance program for people sixty-five or older, younger people with certain disabilities, and people of any age with end-stage renal disease (ESRD). You can find valuable information on options, agencies to contact, and how to change coverage at https://www.medicare.gov.

Note that new enrollees and all covered Medicare participants have a window each year from October 15 through December 7 to change their Medicare health or prescription drug coverage. Once that time passes, the individual must wait until the following year to make changes. Medicare comprises four different parts:

1. **Medicare Part A (Hospital Insurance)** helps cover:
   - Inpatient care in hospitals
   - Skilled nursing facility care
   - Hospice care
   - Home health care
2. **Medicare Part B (Medical Insurance)** helps cover:
   - Services from doctors and other healthcare providers
   - Outpatient care

- Home health care
- Durable medical equipment
- Some preventive services

3. **Medicare Part C (Medicare Advantage):**
   - Includes all benefits and services covered under Part A and Part B
   - Usually includes Medicare prescription drug coverage (Part D) as part of the plan
   - Run by Medicare-approved private insurance companies
   - May include extra benefits and services for an extra cost

4. **Medicare Part D (Medicare prescription drug coverage):**
   - Helps cover the cost of prescription drugs
   - Run by Medicare-approved private insurance companies
   - May help lower your prescription drug costs and help protect against higher costs in the future

For more information on medical and long-term care insurance, see the "Financial" section of *Eldercare 101.*

OTHER TYPES OF HEALTH COVERAGE

Medicaid

As outlined in the "Financial" section, this is a federally aided, state-operated program that provides medical care for certain low-income individuals and families with limited financial resources. Qualification for this program varies from state to state and depends on marital status. Accessing Medicaid while you receive SSI benefits does not preclude individuals from this program, but some of the SSI benefits will go toward medical costs. Medicaid reimburses 100 percent of medical expenses, other than your SSI deductions. For more detailed information, review your state's Medicaid website or the national Medicaid website at https://www.medicaid.gov.

Veterans Aid & Attendance Benefits

Veterans and their families also should know about the U.S. Department of Veterans Affairs (VA) Aid & Attendance (A&A) benefits. These are benefits paid, in addition to pension, if the veteran requires the aid of another person with ADLs or if the veteran typically pays for assisted-living or a nursing home. Also, in some circumstances, family members of veterans are eligible for health benefits. To determine those circumstances, check out the VA's Civilian and Medical Health Program of Veteran Medical Affairs, Spina

Bifida Program, Children of Vietnam Veterans, Foreign Medical Program, and Caregiver Program. As we note in our "Financial" section of *Eldercare 101*, the nonprofit website, http://www.VeteranAid.org, has great information on who qualifies and how you apply. Additional resources include http://www.benefits.va.gov/insurance, http://www.va.gov/statedva.htm, and http://www1.va.gov/vso/index.asp.

Private Insurance

Private insurance can be purchased by individuals between the ages of eighteen through sixty-five who are still working or were before their circumstances or medical situation prevented them from working. These individuals are covered under individual insurance contracts with specific rules based on the actual plan. There are often co-pays, deductibles, and out-of-pocket annual maximums associated with these healthcare benefits. For more information about private health insurance, check out your state's **SHIBA** program. SHIBA is an organization that protects consumers regarding their health insurance and provides oversight of the insurance industry. Examples of state SHIBA programs can be found at http://www.insurance.wa.gov/ and http://www.oregon.gov/dcbs/insurance/shiba/Pages/shiba.aspx.

Find Out If an Insurance Provider, Doctor, or Local Hospital Offers "Teleservices"

Teleservices include telecare, telehealth, telecoaching, and telemedicine. Elders and their remote caregivers can call or check the Internet for answers to questions about health concerns. These products are often provided through health insurance providers, doctors' offices, and hospitals. Whereas the phone is considered "low tech," these services are important and affordable, often offered as a free "add-on" to health insurances. Elders should check with their insurance company, PCP, or local hospital and ask about what type of phone and Internet support is available.

There's an App for That!

For "virtual" doctor visits, install an app (or go online) and have an online face-to-face "visit" with a doctor to discuss illness symptoms. Search your app store for **Health Express** (by Am Well/Providence).

GERIATRIC DENTISTRY

By Benjamin B. Hellickson, DDS[15]

In the last section, we explored various medical specialties. One in particular, deserves its own subsection: dentistry. Keeping up with oral care is critically important at any age, including during our elder years. But being elderly brings some special considerations regarding oral care:

• Physical, mental, and medical disabilities and diseases
• Adverse reactions to various medications
• Ability to tolerate dental procedures
• Ability to perform adequate oral hygiene
• High prevalence of root caries (cavities)
• Limited financial resources

While no recognized specialty in geriatric dentistry exists, many general dentists find great reward in treating elders. These dentists often will make special accommodations for this patient population—not only in the way the dentists treat an elder's dental and oral needs, but also in the length of time they spend with the patient and in the extra caring manner in which the office personnel treat the older patient.

Read on for a look at how good oral health can translate into good general health. Dr. Ben also explores some of the common oral concerns of elders such as periodontal disease, dentures, and dental implants. He'll close the section with a look at dentistry down the road as well as special dental and oral tips for elders.

THE IMPORTANCE OF GOOD ORAL HEALTH

Research has shown time and time again that proper oral health equates with better general health and, ultimately, quality of life. Because of this direct correlation, elders, encouraged by their families and caregivers, should focus on maintaining good oral health to reduce the potential of acute dental infections and the resulting health complications.

One of the most glaring examples of the need for oral health care in elders is the link between dental plaque and pneumonia. Bacterial plaque, which causes dental infections, spreads pathogens that can cause pneumonia—and pneumonia is the leading cause of death in nursing home patients.[17] There also is a strong correlation between periodontal disease and cardiovascular disease due to the inflammatory nature of periodontal disease. In fact, one study found that patients with periodontitis were 1.6 times more likely to have a stroke.[18]

The good news is that oral health can easily be accomplished through preventative practices. *A regular routine of brushing and flossing, combined with regular dental visits, is still the gold standard for maintaining oral health.* In addition, oral cancer screening is now a common practice among all dentists, and annual oral cancer screening can save lives. If the prevention approach fails—due to inconsistency in the practice, past poor prevention, an accidental tooth crack, or other problems—a properly trained dentist will take a restorative approach to remove caries (cavities) and retain teeth, although damaged teeth may still require extraction to reduce overall bacterial load. Reducing overall bacterial count is a must for aging and vulnerable patients.

Unfortunately, however, this progression is all too common:

Retirement → Decrease of dental insurance → Stop going to dentist → Arthritis and decrease in manual dexterity → Decrease in home care → Increase in bacteria → Increase in active infections (bacterial load) and tooth loss → Painful eating → Decrease in weight due to eating less → Decrease in overall health

One particularly vulnerable elder group is those living in nursing homes. Many nursing home patients are needlessly suffering from dental infections, and they rarely tell anyone about their dental pain unless a dentist is available. We advocate for access to dental care in all nursing homes and highly recommend that nursing home patients who are at high risk for dental infection see a dentist for checkups and treatments *every three to four months*.

COMMON ORAL CONCERNS OF ELDERS

Periodontal Disease

One of the most common oral concerns of elders is periodontal disease, the leading cause of tooth loss. Reportedly, 23 percent of adults over age sixty-five have severe periodontal disease, a chronic inflammation of the tissue that supports the teeth.[19] If teeth are not adequately supported, they will most likely need to be extracted.

Although periodontal disease rates increase as we age, the disease is completely preventable. The magic formula for preventing periodontal disease is:

- Brush after meals and floss once a day before bedtime
- Lower sugar (no soda) intake

• Go for dental cleanings at least twice a year (active infections may require cleanings every three to four months)

Medication Side Effects

Nearly 90 percent of older patients take at least one prescription medication and three over-the-counter drugs each day.[20] And there is a linear relationship between the number of drugs taken and an increase in the potential for adverse drug reactions.

For example, 80 percent of the most commonly prescribed medications cause dry mouth (xerostomia), and 30 percent of people over sixty-five years old suffer from dry mouth (which can also be caused by Sjogren's syndrome and salivary gland radiation). In addition, more than four hundred medications are associated with salivary gland dysfunction.[21]

Oral effects of dry mouth and salivary hypo-function include:

• Dental cavities: Individuals who haven't had a cavity in thirty years can develop new decay with increased dry mouth (especially root cavities, which relate to tooth loss)
• Lack of taste (dysgeusia) and difficulty swallowing (dysphagia)
• Gum inflammation (gingivitis), leading to gum disease (periodontal disease)
• Chewing (mastication) problems
• Fungal infections (candidiasis)
• Poorly fitting dentures

The way to treat problems associated with dry mouth is with:

• High fluoride toothpaste
• Frequent water intake
• Oral moisturizers or lubricants, mouthwashes, and sprays
• Sugar-free gum
• Hard and soft tissue relines of dentures by dentist
• Frequent dental visits (minimum every six months; preferably every three to four months) and x-rays (minimum annually)

There's an App for That!

For those patients and caretakers who are interested in reviewing medications and interactions, **ePocrates Rx** is a great app used by medical and dental professionals (http://www.epocrates.com).

Oncology Considerations

Oncology patients should have a comprehensive dental exam, including x-rays, in advance of surgery and chemotherapy. The goal of the visit is to identify and reduce oral pathogens, thereby eradicating oral disease while the body battles cancer. In essence, optimal oral health leading into cancer treatment will minimize complications.

Dental visit protocol would include:

- Extraction of teeth that cannot be restored or have hopeless periodontal prognosis
- Creation of custom trays for fluoride gels
- A three-month recall schedule for regular cleanings, evaluation, and treatment
- Evaluation of need for 0.12 percent chlorhexidine rinse

Because medications and oral conditions change frequently during cancer treatment, consistent communication between the patient's dentist and her oncologist must take place.

THE LOWDOWN ON DENTURES AND DENTAL IMPLANTS

Despite best efforts, some people will need to have teeth extracted. Having a dentist make a denture is a relatively low-cost means of replacing teeth. Full dentures are for those with no teeth at all, whereas partial dentures can replace as little as one tooth and are supported by existing dentition. A well-fitted, clean denture is a must for maintenance of good overall health.

A properly trained family practice dentist will make great dentures for the average patient. For those patients with more complex oral issues, a *prosthodontist* may be required. However, always start with your elder's preferred general dentist, as there will likely be an existing rapport, and that dentist can "quarterback" all dental treatment.

Once someone has a denture, visits to the dentist are not over. On the contrary, the underlying tissue and bone that supports the denture is constantly changing, which means the fit of the denture will definitely change. In addition to normal changes in anatomy, dentures also can become ill fitting as a result of infection or oral cancer.

Some signs of ill-fitting dentures to watch for include:

- Elder changes eating habits
- Elder stops talking
- Elder stops taking out dentures

Denture adjustments are relatively easy and must also become part of the regular oral health routine.

Denture Loss or Breakage

Most dentures today come from the lab with the *patient's name imprinted on them.* (Ask your dentist if her lab does this.) Despite this loss-prevention practice, it's not uncommon for elders to lose or break their dentures. If this happens, they should replace the dentures as soon as possible.

Success of a new denture after loss or breakage directly correlates to how quickly it is replaced. That is, the rate at which a patient will regularly wear her dentures can decrease by 30–40 percent if the denture is not replaced within three months, and denture loss is tied to overall health decline.

Without her dentures, the elder most likely will find eating uncomfortable, maybe even painful, and stop or minimize eating. Without proper nutrition, serious trouble is just around the corner.

Dental Implants

Although dentures are still the typical means of replacement for missing teeth, dental implants are quickly becoming a much better replacement option and can be used in conjunction with dentures. In fact, implants have success rates in the 90+ percent range!

Multiple implants can be placed, and dentures can snap in on top of these implants either permanently or in a way that dentures can be removed daily for cleaning. By having more secure dentures, patients often more readily adapt and eat better. If your elder needs to have teeth extracted, discuss the pros and cons of dentures and dental implants with her dentist.

DENTISTRY IN THE NEXT TWENTY YEARS

Dentistry has changed drastically during the lifespan of today's elders. Whereas dental care was once scarce and, daresay, painful, it can now not only be painless but also help prolong life. Over the next twenty years, we also can expect more changes to come with respect to this growing population.

Tomorrow's "oldest-old" will:

• Be better educated (overall and dentally)
• Have more of their natural teeth

- Have higher expectations (i.e., more cosmetic dentistry; implants to replace toothless areas instead of dentures)
- Be in need of more complex dental treatment
- Be in need of dentists with a broader medical understanding and willingness to treat medically complex patients

Here are some examples of new technology and procedures coming down the road that will continue to improve the oral and, ultimately, overall health of our elders:

- **Intraoral scanners:** This technology scans teeth needing crowns and transmits the data to a lab for crown fabrication, eliminating the need for uncomfortable impressions.
- **Same-day crowns:** Intraoral scanners can transmit a scan of the tooth needing a crown to an in-office milling machine, which mills the crown in approximately one hour. This eliminates the need for patients to come back the following week to have the crown seated.
- **Dental lasers:** New technology is being developed and improved for use in gum surgery, in stopping bleeding during procedures, and in deep cleaning.
- **More comfortable dental chairs:** Although comfortable chairs may seem like a small luxury, the importance of keeping patients comfortable while undergoing checkups and procedures contributes to a better overall experience.
- **Mobile dental offices:** RV-type vehicles are being retrofitted into dental offices that can contract with nursing homes and other elder facilities to provide care for immobile patients.

TIPS FROM THE DENTIST

The Daily Routine of Oral Hygiene

Use an electric toothbrush: As aging patients lose manual dexterity and arthritis sets in, electric toothbrushes make regular brushing much easier. A few of the popular brands include Sonicare and Oral B. They can be expensive, but ask the dentist if she can offer them at a discount. Also, the replacement heads are expensive as well, but stores regularly offer coupons to make purchasing them less cost prohibitive.

Stuck on a manual toothbrush? Twinbrush is a duel-headed toothbrush which promotes the Bass Method of cleaning at the gumline and saves time. Search online for "Bass Method of teeth brushing" to view a number of YouTube videos demonstrating the technique.

For patients who have a hard time holding a toothbrush: Wrap tape or an elastic bandage around the handle. A sponge or rubber grip attached to the handle are other options for facilitating a better hold.

Use oral rinses for dry mouth: Biotene and Carifree, in particular, have a line of oral rinses and gels.

Xylitol gum: This gum increases saliva flow and neutralizes pH in the mouth.

Picks, flossers, and tongue brushes: Ask the dentist about the array of dental tools on the market designed to aid home oral care. She even may have samples for you!

Before the Dentist Appointment

Who to choose: As "corporate" dentistry increases, elders should carefully consider their choice of dentist. Although great dental care can be had at a corporate dental office, corporate dental models tend to have a higher turnover rate and may not offer the consistency and familiarity for an elderly patient that a private or group practice can offer.

Request an extended exam: Dentists should be willing to take more time with elderly patients. When calling for an appointment, request an extended exam. Dentists and staff will appreciate the advance warning.

Inform your dentist of the following:
1. High blood pressure on the day of treatment
2. Use of bisphosphonates (medications to prevent the loss of bone mass or to treat osteoporosis and similar diseases)
3. Recent stroke (should delay more extensive treatment such as extractions for at least six months)
4. Acute infection (makes it difficult to anesthetize)
5. Use of anticoagulants (inform dentist of medication and, if appropriate, get a PT/INR). The prothrombin time (PT) and its derived measures of prothrombin ratio (PR) and international normalized ratio (INR) are measures of the extrinsic pathway of coagulation. This test is also called "ProTime INR" and "PT/INR." Communication of a current PT/INR to staff, family, and doctors may lead to an adjustment of medications that could be life-saving.

Final Tip: WebMD has a great page on frequently asked questions for the elderly dental patient: http://www.webmd.com/oral-health/guide/senior-dental-care-faq.

THE AGING BODY

Thus far in this section of *Eldercare 101*, we have covered medical topics pertaining to elders who, for the most part, care for themselves with minimal support from you or another caregiver. But when the balance of wellness tips to the point when someone is unable to leave home or care for herself, then it is helpful to understand in what particular areas that person needs care and to determine the appropriate course of action or support.

In this section, we will explore various options and progressive stages of medical support services.

MEDICAL IMPLANTS FOR THAT SECOND LEASE ON LIFE

According to the CDC, one in three elders has two or more chronic conditions.[21] Thanks to significant medical advances, even in just the last two decades, many of these conditions can be managed with the help of exciting new medical technologies. Here's a list of some of those implants and devices that can potentially be life-saving or life-enriching—offering elders a second lease on life:

Cochlear Implant: A cochlear implant is a small, complex electronic device that can help to provide a sense of sound to a person who is profoundly deaf or severely hard of hearing. This is different from a hearing aid, as the cochlear implant bypasses damaged portions of the ear and directly stimulates the auditory nerve.

Corneal Implant: A damaged or diseased cornea can be replaced with donated corneal tissue, either entirely or partially, through a surgical procedure.

Defibrillator: An implantable cardioverter defibrillator (ICD) is a small device placed in the chest or abdomen. Doctors use the device to help treat irregular heartbeats called arrhythmias. An ICD uses electrical pulses or shocks to help control life-threatening arrhythmias, especially those that can cause sudden cardiac arrest.

Dental Implant (also known as an endosseous implant or fixture): This is a surgical component that interfaces with the bone of the jaw or skull to support a dental prosthesis such as a crown, bridge, denture, or facial prosthesis or to act as an orthodontic anchor. (See previous section on dentistry and care.)

Hip Replacement: Age increases the incidence of osteoarthritis, which causes joint pain. One alternative to the pain is undergoing a surgical procedure in which the hip joint is replaced by a prosthetic implant.

Knee Replacement: Knee replacement surgery is a surgical procedure in which the knee joint is replaced by a prosthetic implant.

Pacemaker: This small device, when surgically placed in the chest or abdomen, helps to control arrhythmias (abnormal heart rhythms). This device uses electrical pulses to prompt the heart to beat at a normal rate.

Transvaginal Mesh (recalled in January 2012): This net-like implant is used to treat pelvic organ prolapse and stress urinary incontinence in women. The product design and implantation technique, however, contributed to serious complications such as erosion and organ perforation. The product, thus, has been recalled, and the procedure is banned. Some elders still have transvaginal mesh, if they did not adhere to the recall and have the mesh removed.

Important Questions: Does your elder have some sort of implant? If yes, what is it, and is there "maintenance" that should be addressed? Also, is it documented in the advance directive with your elder's medical wishes?

WHAT IF I CAN'T LEAVE MY HOME?

Some elders stay healthy enough and have the right kind of support, allowing them to age at home. Even for those individuals, there may come a time when they cannot leave their home to seek medical attention or to pick up a prescription. What are the options for these elders during such circumstances?

Not to fear! If you have a phone, it will come! There are very few services in the twenty-first century that are not available to our elders in their own homes.

Home Health Team

Even PCPs such as MDs, DOs, NPs, and PAs are joining the ranks of healthcare practitioners who will visit, assess, treat, and bill for services in home settings. Most of these individuals bill either under their clinic or office name as a group or individually. Some physician practices offer "concierge services," which bill annually rather than as a fee per service. Note that mobile healthcare practitioners are limited to their skills at hand and are unable to do complicated procedures in the home setting, but just their willingness to travel is helpful for many elders who are unable or unwilling to leave home.

If an elder has an identified skilled need—one of the identified ADLs—then Medicare will pay for skilled services including a home health or hospice team to visit the patient in her home. These teams might include nurses, PTs, OTs, speech therapists, psychiatric nurses, and home health aides. In the case of hospice, all the these skilled services are included in addition to social workers or counselors, hospice physicians, volunteers, and chaplains.

Prescriptions and Medical Equipment/Supplies

More and more companies are delivering prescriptions or medical equipment and supplies either by car or by mail. Some of the supplies and equipment may be covered by insurance, depending upon the insurance program. Some examples of items that can be delivered to the home include but aren't limited to:

• Pharmaceuticals and medical supplies
• Durable medical equipment
• Home oxygen and supplies
• Incontinence and ostomy supplies
• Nutritional and enteral supplies and materials

Under hospice, pharmaceutical and durable medical equipment are also covered by insurance, if they are connected to the diagnosis.

Other In-Home Services and Care Providers

These options were explored in depth in the "Social" section of *Eldercare 101*. As a reminder, know that these in-home services and care providers can potentially enable your elder to age at home, despite medical maladies:

• Housekeepers
• Hourly or shift caregivers
• Art, music, massage, and other therapists
• House manager, chef, and landscape services

Also, food and other household supplies can be delivered, and transportation to and from medical and other appointments is just a click or phone call away!

Beyond Home

If bringing healthcare services into your elder's home is not feasible for any reason (unaffordable, elder is disagreeable, elder is too medically needy, etc.), it may be time to consider other living arrangements such as an adult foster home, CCRC, ALF, memory care facility, nursing home, or skilled nursing facility. These options were described in our "Living Environment" section.

GETTING IN-HOME HEALTH CARE

The areas generally evaluated by medical and long-term health insurance companies to determine if they will pay for home health care are the **ADLs**. They address key areas determining if a person is capable of taking care of herself and include the following:

- **Eating:** Preparing meals and feeding oneself
- **Dressing:** Putting on and taking off clothes of the upper and lower body
- **Grooming:** Brushing teeth, washing face, and caring for hair and skin
- **Bathing:** Washing the entire body on a routine basis, either in tub or shower
- **Toileting:** Getting to and from the toilet and maintaining reasonable personal hygiene
- **Ambulating:** Moving around within one's living space
- **Transferring:** Moving from sitting to standing, including in and out of a bed or chair with or without the use of adaptive devices or supports

If your elder is unable to do any of these listed ADLs, she may need support with:

- Preparing meals
- Shopping
- Housework and laundry
- Getting to appointments
- Paying bills and other money matters
- Home maintenance and repair
- Using the phone
- Taking medication as prescribed (including insulin, oxygen, and eye, ear and on-the-skin medication)
- Treatments prescribed by the PCP (including colostomy, bladder catheters, wound care, etc.)

Notice that some of the needs are "custodial" in nature and some are "medical" in nature. In the section on "In-Home Helpers" in the "Living Environment" section of *Eldercare 101*, we discuss finding in-home *custodial* help. However, if your elder needs *medical* help, the PCP would refer your parent to a home healthcare agency.

Through a home healthcare agency, a registered nurse (RN), social worker, certified nursing assistant (CNA), personal care aide (PCA), or home health aide (HHA) would visit your elder at home and make an effort to cure or treat your elder's illness or injury. The healthcare worker also might teach your elder how to use a new adaptive device for a limited period of time. Examples of some of the work that home healthcare providers offer include:

- Ongoing IV therapy for pain management, cancer, or the like
- Skilled wound care
- Training for a new ostomy or catheter
- Personal care such as bathing
- Medication management

Insurance Note: The fees of home health caregivers may or may not be covered by Medicare or Medicaid. To qualify for LTC reimbursement for home health care, an elder must be unable to complete two or three ADLs, depending on her insurance.

FACILITIES BEYOND THE HOSPITAL WITH MEDICAL EXPERTS

Whether your elder is living at home, at an ALF, or at an adult foster home, if her health is such that she needs skilled nursing care but not hospitalization (and her ALF does not have skilled nurses on staff), she may be directed to one of the following:

Nursing Home: A privately operated establishment providing maintenance and personal or nursing care for persons (elders or the chronically ill) who are unable to care for themselves properly and require *medical* attention.

Skilled Nuring Facility (SNF): The terms *skilled nursing facility* and *nursing home* are often used interchangeably, but they are not the same. If your elder qualifies for intensive care following a stay at a hospital, Medicare will only pay for a SNF. The guidelines for qualifying as a SNF require a higher number of skilled nurses and doctors than a nursing home. However, many, if not most, nursing homes do qualify as SNFs. You can acquire a list of certified facilities in your area from your medical insurance provider.

Inpatient Rehabilitation Facility (IRF): Similar to nursing homes, these facilities provide doctor-ordered medical care for people who have suffered an injury or illness, no longer need to be in the hospital, but are unable to return home because they need intensive rehabilitative therapy. IRFs typically provide therapy several hours a day, and the patient must be medically stable enough to handle that level of rehabilitation. Such an intensive level of therapy usually is not available at many SNFs or nursing homes; SNFs can be an interim step for patients who need skilled nursing care but are not yet ready for acute rehabilitation. In essence, patients can use the SNF step to gain strength before moving to the IRF. The discharge planner at the local hospital is the best resource for IRFs in the community.

Digging Deeper

Some ALFs and CCRCs offer nursing services for those residents who need regular medical attention. For more information on ALFs and CCRCs, see the "Living Environment" section. To find nursing homes, skilled nursing facilities, and rehab facilities in your community—and to compare them—check out this Medicare link: http://www.medicare.gov/nursinghomecompare/search.html.

MEDICARE AND INPATIENT CARE IN A FACILITY

Medicare Part A covers two types of inpatient nursing and rehabilitation care, under different rules and limitations as described next. Medicare, however, does not cover long-term nursing home residence, or a stay of any length in a nursing facility for *custodial* care, or any level of care that doesn't meet all the following Medicare-set conditions.

Skilled Nursing Facility

- Patient's stay must begin *within thirty days of a hospital stay of at least three days*.
- Patient must need and have a physician's prescription for daily skilled nursing care or physical rehabilitation.
- Care must be in a Medicare-certified SNF.
- Coverage lasts only while the patient's condition is improving. Once the patient's condition has stabilized, Medicare Part A will no longer cover inpatient care.

Inpatient Rehabilitation Facility

- Patient must need and have a physician's prescription for acute rehabilitation consisting of *at least two different types of therapy* (e.g., PT *and* SLP, or PT *and* OT). Patient must need and have a physician's prescription for *at least three hours* of rehab therapy.
- Patient must need to receive the rehab care as an inpatient as prescribed by a physician and justified by the facility on an ongoing basis.
- Care must be in a Medicare-certified IRF.

- Coverage lasts only as long as the patient needs the qualifying level of care.
- No prior hospitalization is necessary.

What Medicare Pays

Skilled Nursing Facility

Day 1–20: Medicare Part A pays the full Medicare-approved amount for the cost of a SNF day during one benefit period. A benefit period is the period during which someone is a hospital inpatient, plus the following period in a Medicare-covered SNF or IRF. A benefit period begins on the first day in the hospital and continues until the patient has been out of the hospital and any other Medicare-covered nursing or rehabilitation facility for sixty consecutive days.

Day 21–100: Medicare Part A pays the full Medicare-approved amount during any one benefit period, except for a daily co-insurance amount of $161 per day (as of 2016), within the benefit period.

Day 100 Plus: Medicare no longer pays any of the cost.

Inpatient Rehabilitation Facility

Medicare pays 100 percent of Medicare-approved amount for the stay for as long as Medicare agrees the inpatient care is medically necessary.

TRANSITION TIME

Transitions in care can be challenging. That is, moving from the hospital to a skilled nursing facility, or from home to an ALF, or just coming home from a long procedure at the PCP's office can be exhausting and overwhelming. Such transitions can mean changes in medication, new treatments, or need for follow-up appointments with other healthcare providers.

Points to remember and to help make the transition flow more smoothly:

- **Ask unanswered questions before leaving:** Easily reaching the person who wrote the discharge instructions will be nearly impossible once you and your elder say good-bye.
- **Clarify regarding follow-up appointments:** If one is requested, know whom the appointment is with and whether or not the appointment has already been scheduled. If it hasn't, what is the contact information? If a follow-up appointment has been made, ask for the number to call if your elder needs to reschedule for any reason.

- **How to handle reactions or worrisome symptoms:** Your elder should be provided with a list of signs and symptoms that will warrant a phone call to a PCP (e.g., fever, swelling of an extremity, pain that lasts for more than two hours after taking pain medication). Be sure to know what number to call if you have concerns and ask if they take calls twenty-four hours a day, seven days a week. If they do not, ask for an on-call, backup phone number that will accept your questions twenty-four/seven.
- **How to handle prescriptions:** If your elder is given prescriptions to fill, call the pharmacy first before leaving your current location and ensure they have the medication you will be filling. Often, the prescription can be faxed ahead to the pharmacy, and then they will fill the prescription once you walk in the door to pick up the medication. Ask the pharmacy staff their hours and what they need in order to fill the new prescription (e.g., insurance card, money for a co-pay, and someone to whom to give instructions).
- **Treatment instructions:** If a treatment has been prescribed, ensure someone has provided you or someone on your elder's healthcare team detailed instructions, timing of that treatment, and necessary supplies. Review the instructions, and let the PCP or healthcare provider know if your elder is unable to perform any of the treatments prescribed; she may need assistance. **Tip:** Getting the help of staff from a home health agency can take up to seventy-two weekday hours in some areas! This can delay needed treatments if not thought through, so take this into account when agreeing to discharge to the next place.
- **Questions after getting home:** Some primary and healthcare providers will call the elder at home the following day to ensure the transition is going smoothly. Write down any questions, so they can be asked when the phone call is received.
- **Update!** Using the discharge instructions, compare and update medication and diagnosis lists as well as your elder's record of medical visits.

Simple, downloadable **"Diagnosis List"** and **"Record of Medical Visits"** forms can be found at https://rowman.com/ISBN/9781442265462.

PROFESSIONAL HELP DURING TRANSITIONS

In making the transition from a hospital stay to home or a facility, from home to a facility, or from one facility to another, a number of professionals may be involved and helpful:

Aging Life Care Managers: Aging experts who work with older adults and their adult children and loved ones to develop holistic aging plans and programs addressing all aspects of aging. They are advocates for elders and caregivers. As "age navigators," their primary goal is to define an approach to aging that supports maximum capable independence for the elder. Typically, ALCMs have a health, social services, or gerontology background and most hold advanced degrees. See http://www.aginglifecare.org.

Case Managers: These individuals work for insurance companies. Their main role is to interpret and apply the benefits of that insurance to its members. They often have large caseloads of members to advocate for and support.

Discharge Planners: Professionals whose role is to facilitate an effective and appropriate discharge from the hospital to home or another setting. They work with insurance case managers and other healthcare providers in the hospital to ensure a smooth transition from hospital to home, nursing home, or another community setting.

Finance or Billing Advocates: These individuals work in the area of finance and billing. They can coordinate with insurance case managers to facilitate the accurate accounting of healthcare charges and assist with interpreting your elder's healthcare bills. They also can advocate on your elder's behalf regarding billing within her particular health system.

Nurses at the PCP's Office: These health professionals coordinate care determined by the primary care provider. They often work with insurance case managers and other community healthcare providers.

Resource Coordinators: These individuals are hired by a healthcare system to advocate for and help patients navigate their system. They also can suggest and connect your elder with community resources for support and education. Large healthcare systems will hire individuals to advocate for large numbers of people at a time.

For a downloadable form to keep track of your elder's **"Transition Gurus,"** go to https://rowman.com/ISBN/9781442265462.

AGING LIFE CARE MANAGERS TO THE RESCUE!

As noted numerous times throughout *Eldercare 101*, an ALCM is a health and human services care professional who helps older adults and their families navigate the healthcare system, advocates on the part of the individual client, and works toward common goals of independence and safety. ALCMs come from a variety of healthcare backgrounds such as gerontology, nursing, and social work. These professionals have extensive training and background with a specialized focus on issues associated with aging and disabilities. Through consultation, assessment, care coordination, and advocacy, an ALCM offers specific crisis management, care planning and management, situational consulting, and emotional support to elders and their families.

The Association of Aging Life Care Managers (formerly called the National Association of Professional Geriatric Care Managers) was formed in 1985 to advance dignified care for older adults and their families. They assist older adults who wish to remain in their homes, or can help families in the search for a suitable nursing home placement or extended care if the need occurs. They also maintain a database on their website so that others can find a care manager in their area. Check out http://www.aginglifecare.org.

You can expect ALCMs to meet with you initially to clarify your goals and expectations, discuss the variety of services they offer, set an appointment to assess the elder in mind, and create a comprehensive plan of care. Once the plan of care is developed and agreed upon, the frequency and length of visits will be determined to meet the needs of the elder. Typically, ALCMs will work with an elder from initiation of services until her death or other transition (e.g., move to another state). She also will provide a smooth transition to another ALCM if that is prudent and realistic. You can expect an ALCM to offer an agreement in writing that describes her fees and what services will be provided.

In general, an ALCM's **Initial Assessment** will address the following:

- **Physical Assessment** of health history and physical signs and symptoms, as well as a review of body systems, medications, chronic and current conditions and treatments, nutrition and its effect on function, and other healthcare providers.
- **Social/Emotional Assessment** of social support system (including family and friends), family values and preferences, life satisfaction, stress level and coping mechanisms, mood, history of behavioral or emotional problems, coping mechanisms, substance abuse, and sleep patterns or disturbances.
- **Functional Assessment** of ADLs, assistive devices used to perform ADLs, level of assistance required, and a description of who provides the assistance and for what duration.
- **Spiritual Assessment** of religious beliefs and support systems; personal, religious, or mystical symbols, icons, or treasures; and lists of personal prayers, songs, and stories.

• **Home Safety Evaluation** of architectural barriers, physical and health barriers, structural and design strengths, and need for interior and exterior home modifications.

The ALCM's **Plan of Care** will provide a variety of other suggestions and recommendations such as:

• **Community Resources:** Other individuals, healthcare providers, and associations in the community that can offer support, advice, and education.
• **Suggested Plans of Action:** Recommendations of action, appointments, and directions to consider for the elder and the family.
• **Advocacy:** The ALCM may accompany the elder (and a family member) to healthcare appointments, or urgent and emergency visits.
• **Education:** Provides education and information that is beneficial for the overall health and wellness of the client and her family.

ELDERS AND THE WORLD OF BRAIN DISEASE

Many older adults and the adults who care for them seek medical services because of physical or mental changes. These changes can occur quickly or slowly over time. Most physical changes can be easy to see and address. Mental changes, however, can be more challenging because they aren't as visible and because individuals can function differently at times, making a diagnosis difficult to pinpoint. Mental changes also can be triggered by a physical malady such as a urinary tract infection, so seeking medical help in getting to the bottom of mental changes is critical. Visits to specialists such a geriatric psychiatrist, neurologist, or psychiatric nurse practitioner for assessment would be warranted.

This section will examine some of the most common brain diseases and disorders affecting elders. Knowing what is occurring can help to determine what support and resources to seek.

WHAT IF IT'S A MENTAL ISSUE?

As one grows older, conditions such as dementia, depression, and stroke can disturb one's ability to function or cope. As they struggle to comfort their loved one, family members often feel helpless when it comes to mental health issues. Unfortunately, mental health diseases are widely underrecognized and undertreated. Many mental illnesses in elders are assumed to be side effects of medications or treatments. Most importantly, mental illness is not a normal part of aging.

Generally, if Mom becomes unable to care for herself, you, as the loving advocate, need to work with your parent's PCP to determine a course of action. If Uncle Ted is diagnosed with mild cognitive impairment, medication is only one step of treatment. At this stage, the home healthcare team might expand to include a mental health nurse or a mental health NP. Psychiatric NPs, psychologists, and psychiatrists also can meet with and treat elders one-on-one.

The journey of mental illness is never easy, and it can be made many times worse if family members do not have the tools to take care of their loved ones—as well as themselves. An ALCM would be a great resource to help you determine how your family will care for your elder if dementia or another form of mental illness is the diagnosis. Your options may be:

- Keep your elder **at home with twenty-four/seven monitoring and care** (depending upon severity of cognitive impairment).
- Move her to an **ALF or CCRC that has a memory care unit**, so she can stay at the facility as her dementia worsens.
- Move her to a **designated memory care facility**.

Another option, if ongoing medication and therapy do not successfully manage your elder's mental issues, is to admit her to a **psychiatric facility**. In some states, there are specialized psychiatric hospitals for older adults called **geriatric psychiatry hospitals**. In other states, some facilities have a few beds licensed and set aside specifically for elders. The general admitting criteria often include the following:

- Sixty-five years and older
- Threatened the safety of self, others, or property
- Talked about or tried committing suicide
- Acted in a way that interferes with caregivers' ability to care for her
- Has symptoms that are difficult to diagnose or treat in a doctor's office or other outpatient setting
- Said she does not want help, even though her health and safety may be in danger

DIAGNOSIS DEMENTIA

Dementia is a chronic or persistent disorder of the mental processes marked by memory disorder, personality changes, impaired reasoning, and the like due to brain disease or injury. Although various types of dementia with different symptoms and prognoses are known, in general, as dementia progresses and worsens, the individual's ability to communicate may become impaired before physical changes are noticed.

Location Monitoring: There's an App for That!

One of the most challenging aspects of dementia is wandering and getting lost. Luckily, GPS is available on most smartphones, smart watches, and other wearable technology. With such technology, if a person is missing, care providers or others with authorized access to the technology can locate the elder.

Check your elder's phone for information on how to share her location with others. She also may have a phone setting that, if selected, an alert will be sent to your cell phone maker if her cell phone battery is dangerously low. This will allow a last signal to be sent before the battery dies, and this information can be shared with law enforcement, if needed.

In addition, apps that would be extremely helpful include **Circle of 6** and **Find My Friends** for Apple and Android users. At the click of a button you can see if your elder is at the local grocery store—or on her way to Hawaii!

There are a variety of dementias, although recent research is now showing that over 50 percent of individuals have mixed dementias. Here is a list of some of the known dementias:

- **Alzheimer's:** Dementia that causes problems with memory, thinking, and behavior. Symptoms usually develop slowly and get worse over time, becoming severe enough to interfere with daily tasks. Prognosis varies between four and twenty years.
- **Parkinson's:** A decline in thinking and reasoning often develops in someone diagnosed with Parkinson's disease at least a year earlier.
- **Vascular:** Occurs as multi-infarct or post-stroke dementia. It is less common than Alzheimer's as a sole cause of dementia.
- **Lewy Body:** Dementia that also includes disorders with movement symptoms such as hunched posture, rigid muscles, a shuffling walk, and trouble initiating movement.
- **Creutzfeldt-Jakob:** A rare and rapidly fatal dementia that impairs memory and coordination and causes behavior changes.
- **Other Dementias:** Frontotemporal, primary progressive aphasia, Pick's disease, and progressive supranuclear palsy.

If you see any of the following behavioral changes, your elder might be experiencing mental health changes resulting in a dementia or other brain disease. She will need assessment and, most likely, increased care and support:

- Wandering from home at unusual or unreported times
- Overall mood and personality appear different, sometimes different at a time of day
- Attitude is different without an apparent reason (such as loss or grief)
- Repeats questions, often with information that has just been explained
- Unable to recognize something or someone familiar
- Refuses to participate in personal care and grooming
- Refuses to eat, eats significantly less portions, or eats inedible things
- Becomes demanding and irritable without cause
- Starts hoarding or gathering things with no apparent reasons
- Walks from room to room, in the same pattern, day or night, for no obvious reason
- Unable to care for home, personal belongings, pets, or spouses or partners
- Other unusual behaviors not part of this individual's history or background

Resources to Turn to for More Information

http://www.Alz.org
http://www.nia.nih.gov/alzheimers/vascular-dementia-resource-list
http://www.scie.org.uk/publications/dementia/resources/

ALZHEIMER'S DISEASE

Alzheimer's disease is the most common form of dementia. It is a progressive disease that worsens over time and in the severity of its symptoms. Older adults have difficulty remembering certain things as they age, however, those with Alzheimer's disease have progressive and severe memory loss that is most pronounced with new information, confusion, and changes in mood and personality.

According to the Alzheimer's Association website, the ten warning signs of Alzheimer's disease are:

1. Memory loss that disrupts daily life
2. Challenges in planning or solving problems
3. Difficulty completing familiar tasks at home, at work, or at leisure
4. Confusion with time or place
5. Trouble understanding visual images and spatial relationships

6. New problems with words in speaking or writing
7. Misplacing things and losing the ability to retrace steps
8. Decreased or poor judgment
9. Withdrawal from work or social activities
10. Changes in mood and personality

Alzheimer's disease is prevalent in the United States in the following ways:

- More than five million Americans are living with the disease.
- Approximately five hundred thousand people are dying each year because they have Alzheimer's.
- One in three elders dies with Alzheimer's or another form of dementia.
- Alzheimer's is the sixth leading cause of death in the United States.
- It's the only cause of death among the top ten in America that cannot be prevented, cured, or even slowed.

And women are at the epicenter of the epidemic:

- In her sixties, a woman's lifetime risk for developing Alzheimer's is one in six. For breast cancer, it's one in eleven.
- Almost two-thirds of Americans with Alzheimer's are women.
- There are 2.5 times more women than men providing care twenty-four/seven for someone with Alzheimer's.
- More than 60 percent of Alzheimer's and dementia caregivers are women.

See the **Alzheimer's Association's** helpful website at http://www.Alz.org, where you can access lots of information about the disease including the flyer "Know the 10 Signs: Early Detection of Alzheimer's Disease," that goes into depth about each warning sign. There you can also find out if your community has a local chapter with support groups specifically for the caregivers of those with Alzheimer's.

PARKINSON'S DISEASE

Another degenerative brain disorder is Parkinson's disease. Parkinson's progresses slowly in most people. Initially, it is characterized by unconscious movement of the face and hands, followed by muscular rigidity with progressive changes. After someone has been diagnosed with Parkinson's for a while, the disease can devolve into a decline in reasoning and thinking. Most people's symptoms, however, take years to develop, and they live for years with the disease.

According to the National Parkinson Foundation website, the ten warning signs of Parkinson's include:

- Tremor or shaking
- Small handwriting
- Loss of sense of smell
- Trouble sleeping
- Trouble moving or walking
- Constipation
- A soft or low voice
- Masked (serious-looking, blank stare) face
- Dizziness or fainting
- Stooping or hunching over

In the United States, 50,000–60,000 new cases of Parkinson's disease are diagnosed each year, adding to the one million people who currently have Parkinson's. The CDC rated complications from Parkinson's disease as the fourteenth leading cause of death in the United States. Worldwide, it is estimated that four to six million people suffer from the condition.

For more information about Parkinson's disease, see the website of the National Parkinson Foundation at http://www.parkinson.org. Your community may have a local chapter with support groups.

THIRTEEN TIPS FOR DEMENTIA CAREGIVERS

By Marguerite Manteau-Rao, LCSW, ATR
Author of *Caring for a Loved One with Dementia:*
A Mindfulness-Based Guide for Reducing Stress and
Making the Best of Your Journey Together
www.presencecareproject.com

1. Start your day with a few minutes of mindfulness practice, and end the same way.
2. Incorporate mindfulness into your routines: walking, doing chores, or caring for loved one.
3. Practice recognizing and being with your emotions, including difficult ones.
4. Practice loving kindness for yourself, and also for your loved one.

5. Share your mindfulness practice with at least one other care partner.
6. Put your emotions out, either in writing, collages, or other expressive art forms.
7. Share your joys and struggles with other care partners such as you.
8. Get others to help you.
9. Get enough sleep, eat well, and exercise.
10. Validate the person's reality.
11. Still see the person as a whole person, and behave accordingly.
12. Meet the person's five universal emotional needs. Regardless of their cognitive, emotional, or physical state, human beings all have five universal emotional needs: (1) to be needed and useful, (2) to have the opportunity to care, (3) to love and be loved, (4) to have self-esteem boosted, and (5) to have the power to choose.
13. View the person's difficult behaviors as expressions of unmet needs.

Copyright © 2016 by Marguerite Manteau-Rao. Reprinted with permission.

The **Presence Care Project** is an innovative mindfulness-based dementia care training for family and professional care partners (caregivers). Unlike other forms of training that are skills-based only, the Presence Care approach results in sustained attitudinal changes aimed at benefiting care partners throughout the long journey of dementia. Check out their website at http://www.presencecareproject.com.

WHAT TO EXPECT AT THE END

Any review of elders, their health, wellness, and medical care in later years must also include a discussion of death. As we recommend preparing for and proactively facing health issues, so do we recommend contemplating and preparing for death. Considerations in this regard might include where your elder prefers to die, if she wishes to have care teams for support, and how she can fully live every moment until she dies. Whereas we explore these topics in this section from a medical view, they also will be discussed in our "Spiritual" section.

END-OF-LIFE DECISIONS

Individuals who have faced treatment for a disease such as cancer have fought valiantly, endured endless doctor and specialty appointments, and weathered lab tests and having indices checked at frequent intervals. At some point during the process, your elder may weary of the trajectory and wonder whether the effort is worthwhile. For others, the disease progression can be like a roller coaster, but with the ride dipping down further and further at each turn and bend. The ultimate question often becomes: How much is enough? When do I stop treatment and "let nature take its course"?

A good resource if you find yourself in this scenario with your elder is her PCP. The PCP can bring family members and the elder together to discuss various options. Sometimes the question the PCP asks is not, "Should we stop the treatment?" but rather, "If X, Y, or Z occurs, what do you want to do?" For example, pneumonia (infection of the lung and lung tissue) is often a trigger for such a conversation. If the older adult has suffered many infections, there is history to help shape the discussion.

Now is also when having the POLST form filled out really comes into play. As noted in a variety of places throughout *Eldercare 101*, the POLST highlights the wishes of the elder when it comes to emergencies and potentially life-threatening situations. Although it varies from state to state, generally, the form has boxes to check, indicating whether the patient should or should not have cardio-pulmonary resuscitation (CPR), tube feeding, and other medical interventions. As a portable medical order that transfers from one setting to another with the patient, it is intended to give healthcare providers immediate information about what interventions should or should not be undertaken at the end of life or during a life-threatening situation.

These conversations are not easy to have with your beloved elder, but they make it possible for her to stay in charge of her life until the very end, taking off some of the pressure you might feel as her caregiver.

Digging Deeper

A great resource to explore this topic further is Dr. Atul Gawande's book, *Being Mortal: Medicine and What Matters in the End*. Also, be sure to refer to Fr. Larry's discussion in the "Death Dialogue" section within our "Spiritual" chapter.

WHERE TO DIE: HOME VERSUS HOSPITAL AND SPECIAL FACILITIES FOR THE DYING

Home: Most adults prefer to live at home (be it their long-time home, their adult foster home, or their ALF) until they die[22]—and that is entirely possible given the availability of in-home health practitioners and resources. Unless there are other medical reasons for being admitted to a hospital, the PCP can "prescribe" the appropriate team members and services to support your elder at home.

Hospital: If your elder has expressed a desire for and identified in the POLST form life-saving treatments or "full code" in the event of an illness or life-threatening event, then she most likely will be transferred to a hospital for care. If she recovers, she can return home or may need to seek skilled nursing care at a nursing home, SNF, or acute rehabilitation facility, as outlined earlier in this chapter.

Hospice: When your elder's health reaches the point where the end is imminent, her PCP can prescribe hospice care. Generally, once enrolled in hospice, a patient is usually administered care in the home by a team of visiting hospice professionals—with the family caregiver continuing to be the main caregiver. Although hospice can provide round-the-clock care in a nursing home, a specially equipped hospice facility, or, on occasion, in a hospital, this is not the norm. To find hospice agencies in your elder's community, you can use the online agency locator of the National Association for Home Care and Hospice at http://www.nahcagencylocator.com.

Special Inpatient Hospice Facilities: As noted earlier, some communities have inpatient hospice facilities, which provide intensive care at end of life. The staff members at these facilities are specially trained in end-of-life issues and treatment plans. To find an inpatient hospice facility in your area, ask your elder's PCP or ALCM. You can also search online for "hospice facility [plus your city]."

Regarding the few inpatient hospice facilities across the country, be aware that they are all licensed differently. Because of this, the amount of time someone can stay at a particular facility will vary. For example, some small hospitals with inpatient hospice programs only allow patients with symptoms that aren't controllable at home. That means that, if a hospice patient improves, even if she has a terminal diagnosis, she may be forced to return home or to a residential facility that allows a person to stay indefinitely.

HOSPICE CARE

Hospice is a philosophy of care focused on comfort—for the patient and her family—when the patient no longer has curative options or has chosen not to pursue treatment, perhaps because the side effects outweigh the benefits. This comprehensive program, administered through hospice agencies, addresses physical, emotional, and spiritual pain including such common end-of-life concerns as the sense of fear and loss, feeling like a burden, and worrying about the wellbeing of the family left behind. See our "Spiritual" section for more on hospice care and end-of-life approaches.

As noted, hospice care is all encompassing when it comes to end-of-life care and comprises a variety of services and supplies including but not limited to:

- Coordination and care by an interdisciplinary hospice team.
- Durable medical equipment, medications, oxygen, and supplies for pain relief and for treatments related to the life-limiting diagnosis.
- If symptoms are out of control, the hospice staff can authorize to have the elder transferred to a hospital, where care will be provided.
- If the caregivers are in need of rest and support, the hospice team can authorize to have the elder transferred to a nursing facility, where care will be provided.
- Grief and bereavement support for the family following the death of the loved one.
- Occasionally, alternative therapies, depending on authorization from the hospice team.

Hospice Team Members

Hospice Physician: The hospice team "captain," who makes the decision to "accept" someone as a hospice patient and oversees the care. Typically, patients only see the hospice physician once for a face-to-face visit.

Hospice Nurse: Focuses on pain and symptom management and acts as the hospice team "quarterback," communicating with the hospice physician and other hospice team members.

Hospice Aide: Provides assistance with personal care such as showering and bathing, shampooing hair, and other light housekeeping as requested by the client or family. The hospice aide is under the supervision of the hospice nurse.

Hospice Social Worker or Counselor: Focuses on legal, financial, and social issues. She can assist the client and family with end-of-life planning and with communicating with emergency response systems.

Hospice Chaplain: Focuses on spiritual or religious support and intervention and can offer prayer, guided meditation, and other comfort.

Hospice Volunteer: Has been trained for forty hours in how to care for someone who has a terminal illness. She typically visits once per week for four hours to allow the primary caregiver time to run errands or rest, if needed.

What Hospice Team Members Do Not Do

Many families want to know what hospice will do at the very end of life *if your elder is at home.* Will someone from the hospice team stay as long as necessary to care for Mom or Dad in the final days and hours? Will a hospice team member stay up at night so other family members can rest? The answers are, "No." Whereas hospice team members will visit during the day at scheduled times, they do not provide shift care in the home. The hospice nurse and social worker, however, can help you to find around-the-clock caregivers, if needed. Depending upon availability, however, someone from the hospice team is "on call" twenty-four/seven to come to the home in an emergency situation and offer support. An ALCM also can collaborate with and assist the hospice team in addressing end-of-life needs and concerns.

HOSPICE AND MEDICAL INSURANCE

To be eligible for hospice benefits through Medicare:

1. The PCP certifies that your elder has a terminal diagnosis and no more than six months left to live.
2. A hospice physician agrees to the PCP's prognosis.
3. Then Medicare or other insurance will cover hospice benefits (except for the Medicare patient living in a SNF).

Hospice is different from other healthcare services in that hospice agencies charge one cost per patient day. That is, clients are not billed for individual services and visits, because all the services are grouped into one cost and billed a daily fee, which Medicare covers. Medicaid mimics Medicare in its reimbursement of hospice services, and most private insurances do as well. Just to be sure of the details, verify the specific hospice provisions of your elder's medical insurance. You also might check out Medicare's web page on hospice at: http://www.medicare.gov/coverage/hospice-and-respite-care.html.

Also, note that, generally, when someone is covered by insurance for hospice services, the insurance will not pay for:

- Treatments, medications, equipment, and supplies for conditions unrelated to the life-limiting illness
- Care from physicians or other healthcare providers not arranged by hospice
- Room and board if the patient lives at home, in a nursing home, or in a hospice residential facility
- Emergency room visits, inpatient facility care, and ambulance transportation, unless arranged by the hospice team

What Happens When a Patient Is Discharged from Hospice?

An important consideration is that hospice agencies occasionally discharge clients if a patient no longer fits the criteria of having six months or less to live or no longer has the life-limiting diagnosis that qualified her for the hospice services in the first place. If this happens to your elder, she has the right to appeal the decision. To learn how to do so, ask your hospice team or refer to the **National Association of Home Care and Hospice** at http://www. nahc.org. Also know that the insurance rules and regulations regarding someone being discharged from hospice and being able to come back under the program if she requalifies are very complex. Work with your elder's hospice team and insurance provider to understand all the ramifications.

Another Good Resource on Hospice

National Hospice and Palliative Care Organization: http://www.nhpco. org/about/hospice-care

WHAT TO EXPECT WHEN HOSPICE IS RECOMMENDED

PCP Referral: The PCP sends a referral to the chosen hospice agency.

Hospice Agency Review and Initial Processing: The hospice agency reviews the referral. If the hospice physician agrees with the PCP's prognosis, the hospice team verifies insurance benefits, calls the family, and sets up an initial visit.

Initial Visit—The Paperwork: A hospice nurse will facilitate the initial visit. During this visit, the nurse will ask your elder or a family member to sign paperwork authorizing "acceptance of hospice services," which will trigger the ability of the hospice agency to bill your elder's medical insurance; *this agreement also triggers a discontinuation of the insurance company paying for any medical expenses other than what is authorized by the hospice team.*

Initial Visit—The Evaluation: During the initial visit, the hospice nurse also will discuss the available hospice services and—based on her professional evaluation and the input of the patient and her family—identify the hospice team members who will be visiting the patient. In addition, she will determine and order the durable medical equipment, medications, and supplies that will be needed. Each person has different requirements as she reaches life's end. Some people need regular skin and wound care, some choose not to have the chaplain visit, some have enough support that they decline having a volunteer visit for caregiver respite, and others need or request every available hospice service.

Hospice Team Member Visit Arrangements: After the initial evaluation and once the paperwork is signed, start expecting a lot of phone calls. Within two weeks of the initial visit, each team member who was identified as necessary will attempt to call and set up a time to visit your elder. Most hospice team members organize their own schedules, so they will each call individually to arrange meeting times.

Hospice Team Member Visits: The first visit with each hospice service provider might take up to one-and-a-half to two hours, as she gets to know your elder, family members, and caregivers. Follow-up visits usually last approximately thirty to sixty minutes. The frequency of how often each hospice provider visits will depend on the services she provides. You can expect each to review her service plan during the first visit. If you have questions, ask. Also, know that some hospice team members will leave paperwork in the home outlining what they've done during a visit; others use computerized systems and leave synopsis reports at an agreed-upon interval. If all key family members can't be present during every hospice team member visit with your elder and depend upon written communication, discuss the "paperwork trail" with the providers and specify what you would like to see.

Twenty-four/Seven Access for Consultation: If a time comes when your elder is experiencing pain or other symptoms, when you are concerned medications are running out, when your elder is falling or isn't able to get into bed, or when your elder's primary caregiver (perhaps a spouse or you) isn't able to get enough rest, pick up the phone and call the hospice agency—even if the nurse is not scheduled for a visit.

PALLIATIVE CARE

Palliative care is a U.S. board-certified medical specialty focused on keeping a patient comfortable and as pain free as possible. Like hospice, palliative care addresses physical, emotional, and spiritual pain through a comprehensive program that delivers care, symptom treatment, medications, medical equipment, and bereavement counseling. Unlike hospice, however, palliative care is comfort care with or without curative intent. That is, whereas hospice services are specifically geared toward care in the last six months of life, palliative care can be delivered at any time or at any stage during an illness, whether it is terminal or not. For example, when we talk about palliative care, it's often in the context of serious illnesses such as HIV/AIDS, cancer, renal disease, chronic heart failure, progressive neurological conditions, or chronic pulmonary disorders.

For example, with the previously listed conditions, the treating physician would prescribe treatments and medications to address the symptoms, medication side effects, and any pain, depression, or anxiety. She might suggest the patient speak with a counselor or participate in art or music therapy. If the illness causes family stress, a social worker or chaplain might visit with the patient and family members. All these coping mechanisms are considered palliative; they improve the quality of life while coping with an illness.

In addition to differing from hospice care in regard to who is eligible for services (terminally ill versus non-terminally ill) and the timing of those services (last six months of life versus any time), palliative care also differs from hospice care in the care location and what services are included. That is, depending on where your elder lives, palliative care may be administered through a hospital or a regular medical provider, rather than in the home as is the norm for hospice. Also, the services included in the palliative care program can vary from organization to organization. For example, one organization might offer a palliative care team that will visit in the hospital and explain various services that can be provided for your elder when she is discharged from the hospital (home health, community services, etc.). Another organization might be a teleservice that provides phone care consultation.

Another way hospice and palliative care programs differ is in the insurance coverage. Some hospice agencies offer palliative care through the same or different team members and separately bill private insurance or Medicaid; Medicare doesn't currently have an insurance benefit that covers palliative care services at home, although Medicare covers hospice care. Also, unlike hospice, which bills insurance in one lump sum per patient day for all services, each item of inpatient or outpatient palliative care is billed separately. The rules are complex in both cases, so it pays to explore the details of insurance coverage with your elder's insurance company and medical providers when considering hospice or palliative care programs.

Note: There is a national movement encouraging Medicare to offer and provide palliative care services, and we expect to see changes in elder Medicare benefits in the future.

WHAT HAPPENS IN THE FINAL HOURS

Palliative Care at End of Life

Sometimes providing palliative care at the end of life can temporarily disrupt an elder's peace but overall add to comfort. Generally, as symptoms progress and the elder is less aware of her surroundings, the care provided becomes focused on preventing infection and skin breakdown. Care providers are encouraged to turn someone every two hours while awake and every four hours during the night. Basic oral and skin care are attended to, and all are focused on ensuring that the elder isn't in pain, have shortness of breath, or suffer anxiety. Food and fluids are always offered as tolerated (unless the PCP orders otherwise).

One to Two Weeks before Passing:
- Sleeps most of the time. She can awaken, but generally falls back asleep.
- Appetite wanes. Although she may attempt to eat, nothing tastes good anymore.
- There can be disorientation, picking at the sheets or in the air, calling out to others during sleep or during the day.

- Blood pressure is lower than normal.
- Pulse is either slightly faster or significantly slower.
- Temperature of body can either become cooler or hotter.
- Skin changes. She can either be flushed with fever, or cold and bluish from lack of circulation.
- Breathing may increase to twenty to thirty breaths a minute or decrease to nine or six breaths a minute.
- Congestion of the lungs can occur and cause a rattle sound from the upper throat. Sometimes it comes with coughing.

One to Two Days, Maybe Hours, Before the Passing: She might have a surge of energy. All of a sudden the elder might wake up and be able to talk, ask for a favorite food, or request to sit in a favorite chair. Then you might see the following:

- Restlessness can increase because there is less oxygen in the blood.
- Breathing will now be irregular and unpredictable.
- Congestion can become louder and worse when the elder is turned from side to side.
- Face becomes relaxed (if she has good pain control).
- Eyes will open wide, but not as if looking at you. Rather, they are glassy, as if she is looking far away.
- Hands and feet are now more purple or splotchy in color, and cool or cold to touch.
- As time progresses, the elder will not respond to your voice or touch. You should assume she can hear you. Talk and let her know what you are doing, thinking, praying.
- Eventually, the breathing slows down, and the last breath can be followed by one, maybe two very long breaths, sometimes interspersed by no breath.

CARE OF THE BODY AFTER DEATH

There are no specific rules or processes after death. Often, care is determined culturally. (We address after-life arrangements in detail in the "Spiritual" section.) Family members and caregivers can and sometimes do the following, based on the elder's wishes:

- Wash the body
- Remove all medical devices and supplies
- Dress in fresh clothes
- Light candles or dim lighting

- Play soft music
- Offer a drink to toast the elder
- Pray and quietly meditate
- Tell the elder's life stories
- Share in tears and laughter
- Reflect on the impact of the elder's life

Call the Funeral Home or Cremation Service

If hospice is involved, family members can call the hospice agency and the hospice nurse will visit. At this visit, she can call a funeral home or cremation service to arrange for pickup of the body, when the family determines the time is right. If hospice is not involved, a family member will need to call the funeral home or cremation service. Each state varies, but, generally, in many states, the body is allowed to stay at home for twenty-four hours, giving the family time to grieve with the body.

Do We Need to Call the Coroner or Medical Examiner?

Calling the coroner or medical examiner varies depending on where you live and the circumstances of your elder's death. Generally, if the elder is on hospice and death is expected, "cause of death" already has been determined by two medical physicians and involving the coroner or medical examiner is not necessary. If the death is unexpected, however, the funeral home will generally call or ask the coroner to visit and review the body before funeral home staff members take away the body.

What Does the Funeral Home Need to Know?

The funeral or cremation service organization will pick up the body at the time requested by the family. The funeral or cremation service personnel will need to know:

- Full name of deceased
- Date of birth
- Physician's name and cause of death
- If the deceased is an organ donor
- Plans for burial or cremation
- If there are any funeral prearrangements

Follow-up Meeting with the Funeral Home or Cremation Services Director

Depending upon the time of day, the funeral or cremation services director usually sets up an appointment within hours or on the following day to meet with family members. During this time, the funeral or cremation services director will assist the family in writing an obituary or other announcements, in ordering death certificates, and in helping to arrange funeral or memorial services.

CARE FOR EACH OTHER

Even if your elder is on hospice and expected to die, her death can be shocking. Everyone experiences the moment of loss and the time after death differently. There is no wrong or right way to express grief. There just is grief. Here are a few things to consider during this difficult time:

- Watch out for each other. Ensure that the primary caregiver and other family members are drinking water, resting, and eating occasionally.
- Support each other. Allow all family members to express themselves as the unique person each is.
- Encourage the primary caregiver and other family members to take time away from work to handle the various tasks and demands they will have to face.
- Reach out for assistance when needed.
- Accept gestures of help from others including from the professional hospice grief counselors who will follow up with family members after someone's death.

SPIRITUAL PILLAR OF AGING WELLBEING

And while I stood there I saw more than I can tell,
and I understood more than I saw;
for I was seeing in a sacred manner
the shapes of things in the spirit,
and the shape of all shapes
as they must live together like one being.

—Black Elk in *Black Elk Speaks*

Chapter Six

MARY JO'S FIRESIDE CHAT

What Role Does Spirituality Contribute to An Elder's Aging Wellbeing?

The path for an ALCM is rich in the practice of companionship and meaningful encounters with the real. When I look through the lens of spirituality at my role as an ALCM, I find that care navigation is consistently intertwined with spiritual meaning within the priority of quality of life for the elder and his caregivers. I begin by creating a safe space where the spiritual meaning of life and aging may dance together as we jointly lean in to the mystery of meaning in an elder's life and in the caregiver's experience. Through this deep awakening of trust, I can sense how Spirit is moving within the interior landscape of an elder and in the day-to-day activity of his life. During this process, the awareness of deeper relationship with the Divine is imprinted on the elder's soul, whereby meaning and clarity have space to breathe and emerge to nourish and guide his journey.

This exchange is present in every care navigation relationship I have, but one elder comes to mind most clearly. Mary was eighty-four when her adult son, Arman, called me seeking support and advice during a crisis with his mother. Over a two-hour conversation, I journeyed with Arman through what every caregiver must ultimately come to terms with: forgiveness and acceptance. In Arman's case, the journey was to be an accelerated one.

Arman began the conversation with a sigh and heaviness in his voice. I knew immediately I would just listen for a while before gathering the statistical information I needed to help. He explained that his mom had gotten a new dog, Toby, and one day, eight weeks ago, she took Toby for a walk. Toby spotted a cat and lunged, pulling Mary to the ground. Unable to get up and feeling disoriented, Mary laid on the sidewalk for some time until a neighbor came to her rescue. The neighbor wanted to take Mary to the hospital, but Mary refused, saying, "I'm feeling fine. I just need to lie down."

The neighbor walked Mary into her home and left her to rest. Being concerned, she went back to check on Mary a short time later. After ringing the doorbell and getting no response, the neighbor peered through a front window and saw Mary lying motionless on the floor, unconscious. She quickly called the fire department, and, several hours later, Mary was in the intensive care unit on full life support. Mary had filled out her POLST form and stated she wanted life-sustaining measures attempted for a set time.

Fast-forward eight weeks. Mary hadn't awakened from her coma, already had been moved to two different facilities, and needed to make yet another move—this time to a LTC support facility. Her son was emotionally exhausted and searching for the appropriate facility with the rare equipment Mary needed.

During my conversation with Arman, I could see clearly how I would be helping, but the revelation had not yet surfaced for him. After an hour or so, he began to express confusion about how to best support his mom. He and his three brothers wanted to honor her wishes for life support, but the doctors were saying it was unlikely she would recover and her body's systems were slowly shutting down. Arman and his brothers were in the throes of considering taking her off life support. They felt as though it were their decision if she lived or died. This crippling decision led him to call me.

At this point I shifted the conversation to the process of discernment. How do you make this type of decision? Just because medicine can keep a body alive, should that option be chosen? This was a moral issue for this family, and, either way, they would feel the burden of their decision. When we are in the throes of crisis management as caregivers, making any decision without creating internal space to take measure of the situation is challenging. Often, we need a spiritual director or guide to help us center ourselves for this process, and talk it through.

Through his faith tradition, Arman had an understanding of this process. I suggested we look at the decision from this internal space. I first gave him permission to be aware that, no matter what he and his brothers decided, they would feel bad, maybe even guilty. Caregivers have guilt as a constant friend. I know I did when caring for my ninety-two-year-old mother with Alzheimer's disease. I have come to see in my own aging life care management practice that the guilt is more often than not a sign of the great dedication of an individual. As caregivers, we want to give our best at all times—but too often we feel we can never give enough.

Throwing this guilt elephant in the room into the conversation allowed Arman to acknowledge and express all the hidden feelings around his reality.

This alone enabled him to move into a space of self-compassion and gentleness for himself and his brothers. Toward the end of our conversation, Arman was wishing his mom could tell him what to do. I pointed out that her POLST was the place to start, and then to listen to what her body was telling him, because her words were no longer available.

Through this discernment process, Arman and his brothers made decisions over the next week that were right for their family. They decided to bring Mary home and have the three long-distance brothers fly in, allowing them to all be together when they removed Mary from life support. At that point, Mary was immediately put on hospice. She was unable to sustain life for more than a few hours, precious time during which her boys engaged in the process of letting her go.

As an ALCM and a spiritual director, I know that every child of an elder needs a companion to acknowledge, perhaps for the first time, that he is in the process of saying good-bye to an elder, and that he needs forgiveness and compassion on the journey. Some children just need the permission to feel what they are feeling and to be listened to, whereas others need tools and rituals to help them along the way. Most importantly, they need to know they are enough and that they have done their best. Acknowledging that our story eventually and always ends in death makes this acceptance easier.

I know that when I leave a family at the end of a care management session or end-of-life journey, I need to turn over their wellbeing to the stewardship of the Divine as they go on their way. In this process of release, I, in turn, as an ALCM, must be aware of the imprint left on my own heart from companioning through another's story. With intention, I allow for a ritual of sacred space where I can listen to my own internal landscape and breathe. Professional supervision and my own spiritual direction practice also help with this process, but it is equally important for you as a caregiver to have practices that nourish and center your wellbeing.

In the "Spiritual" section of *Eldercare 101*, we address spirituality as a form of wellbeing in elders. I have asked Rev. Larry Hansen to address the hard conversations around death and how to embrace what is coming for all of us. In our culture of denial about death, Father Larry opens the door to show us that spirituality is an important part of our journey that often gets put off until the last minute. As a hospice chaplain for over a decade, Father Larry shares his wisdom on living and dying, and how to have the difficult conversations.

Spirituality and the End(s) of Life

Considerations for the Cared-For and Their Care-Givers

Rev. Lawrence Hansen, BCC/CFHPC, CT

You're going to die. This is a simple truth, one which should need no clarification. But we don't think much about it in our modern world. Perhaps it's because today—as opposed to much of human history—in modern American culture, most people who die are old. Technological advances in medicine have drastically reduced infant, child, and young adult mortality in the United States, and, due to contemporary living patterns and mobility, our elders are too often sequestered in care facilities for the aging. Another complicating factor is that most of us don't grow, raise, or kill the food we eat. We are alienated from the processes that produce our sustenance. Therefore, the natural rhythms of life and death, growth and decay, are foreign to us.

In the current imagination, death is the result of a medical mistake, a tragic oversight, or an unexpected accident. Death is an enemy to be fought rather than an unwanted neighbor who moves in, won't leave, and must be endured, if not fully embraced. But is that the only way to approach the subject?

Dr. Richard Payne, the director of the Duke Institute on Care at the End of Life, has observed that death is not a medical event with spiritual implications, but a spiritual event with medical implications.[1] In this section of our book, with Payne's philosophy in mind, we endeavor to support you in your own reflections about life, its purpose, and its ends—as well as its end.

Please note that any opinions expressed herein are those of the author, not those of either of his employers.

LIVING UNTIL THE END

WHAT IS SPIRITUALITY?

Spirituality is perhaps one of the most misunderstood—or at least misappropriated—words in the English language. Too often, the word is conflated with any number of other terms. In this part of our "Spirituality" section, let's first define what we mean by "spirituality." First, what it's *not*:

- It's *not* morality. Morality has to do with the great "shoulds" and "should nots" found in moral codes: "Do not kill, do not steal, do honor your father and mother." One finds morality codes in just about all civilizations, even though what's "moral" may be understood and fleshed out in widely varying ways. For example, honoring father and mother in many cultures might mean taking them into a child's home when they are old. However, in our modern culture, "honor" might mean to some finding a place for them to live around others of the same age. This brings us to the next "not."
- It's *not* ethics. Ethics has to do with the obligations we owe to one another in our society, as applied to a specific situation. Take the case of a terminally ill person who is only "alive" because machines are breathing for him and circulating blood throughout the body. Is it right or wrong to turn off those machines? After all, we're not supposed to take a life, but is that what we are doing? This is an ethical question.
- It's *not* faith. Faith—which comes from the Latin *fides*, "to trust"—refers to those things in which we have ultimate trust or security. A person might say, "I trust that the universe is ultimately safe and friendly," even though it might not appear so in each individual circumstance. Another person might say, "I trust that Jesus (or the Qur'an) holds the ultimate truth about life."
- It's *not* religion. Religion (from the Latin *religare*, "to bind") refers to the community in which one expresses and observes the rituals and tenets of one's faith, as in "I am a Muslim," or "I am a member of St. Francis of Assisi Church."

At the root of all these "nots" is *spirituality*. According to Christina Puchalski and Betty Ferrell in *Making Health Care Whole*, "Spirituality is the aspect of humanity that refers to the way individuals seek and express meaning and purpose, and the way they experience their connectedness to the moment, to self, to others, to nature, and to the significant or sacred." In essence, spirituality has to do with the ultimate meaning of existence itself. And everyone's spiritual path is unique.

As you consider the scope of your life and not just its end, it's worthwhile to take some time to think about the *ends* of your life: what you see as your purpose, your intention, what life—and, more specifically, *your* life—means to you and what you wish to leave for those who matter to you.

In service of providing the elders for whom you are caring with a structure for spiritual reflection, I will be addressing them directly in this section of *Eldercare 101*. Please share the discussion, exercises, poems, and practices with them. Talk with them about their responses to my thought-provoking questions. Be still and listen to their stories, their wants, and their wishes. Be a loving witness to their life.

CREATING YOUR OWN LEGACY LETTER

In the coming days, begin reflecting on your life. Following are questions that might trigger some insights. Write out those insights, keeping a journal of your reflections. Writing about how you find meaning in your life and what you would like to leave your loved ones in the way of your wishes for them is often referred to as creating your "ethical will," "wisdom will," or "legacy letter."

You don't have to write great essays for this process. Just jot down ideas and insights as they come to you, and then review your entries regularly. You will probably begin to recognize some patterns in your recollections of accomplishments, perceived failures, and everyday thoughts that repeat over time. These will form the core of your reflections and the wisdom you've gained by living. As your ruminations coalesce around central themes, you will see taking shape your own "legacy letter," a gift to yourself as well as your loved ones.

Please note you don't need to wait until the end of your life to reflect upon its meaning. For that matter, whether you're twenty-five or eighty-five, you can't predict when you will die. All you know is that you *will* die, and spending some time considering these large issues is logical.

1. What do you feel has been the purpose of your life?
2. What has given you the deepest sense of accomplishment?
3. Describe who you are and the values and beliefs that directed and defined how you have lived your life.
4. Consider the relationships that have influenced you—the people you hold dear, those close to you, and those you wish were closer.
5. What passions have driven you? What activities or other interests kept you fresh, involved in living, and enjoying life?
6. What are your regrets?
7. What has life taught you that you would like to pass on?

One final note: The document you create at this time in your life will reflect how you see yourself *now*. It's not a static creation. How you see your life and what gives it meaning will certainly continue to evolve as you live into the experiences of the coming years. Plan to revisit and review what you've written regularly—at least once each year—to see what you've gained and perhaps what you need to discard.

Great Resources

For more on legacy letters including samples, check out the beautiful website of **Celebrations of Life** at http://celebrationsoflife.net/ethicalwills. You might also want to create a book or video as a legacy. For ideas and help, check out the services of **Timelines** at http://www.timelines-inc.com.

GIVING IT ALL AWAY

Virtually all the great spiritual traditions counsel against hoarding material possessions. The Hebrew scriptures admonish readers to "not wear yourself out to get rich; be wise enough to desist. When your eyes light upon it, it is gone; for suddenly it takes wings to itself, flying like an eagle towards heaven" (Proverbs 23:4–5). Likewise, in the Christian Gospel, Jesus warns His listeners to "not store up for yourselves treasures on earth, where moth and rust consume and where thieves break in and steal; but store up for yourselves treasures in heaven, where neither moth nor rust consumes and where thieves do not break in and steal. For where your treasure is, there your heart will be also" (Matthew 6:19–20). The Holy Qur'an teaches that, "Your worldly goods and your children are but a trial and a temptation, whereas with God there is a tremendous reward" (64:15). The Second Noble Truth in Buddhism holds that one of the causes of suffering is desire for ephemeral things. Likewise, Hinduism (out of which Buddhism grew) also instructs its adherents not to be attached to material possessions: "When affluence is idolized, it enslaves the individual and lures him away from the meaning and purpose of life."[2] The preachers of the "Prosperity Gospel" notwithstanding, it seems safe to state that no authentic spiritual path encourages the acquisition of material goods as a path to peace and contentment.

On a personal note, my late father was never one for collecting "things." Oh, he had his favorite hunting items and Jim Beam collector bottles; but, other than that, material items didn't seem to hold a lot of interest for him. When asked about this, he would reply with a rhetorical question: "You know why they don't have luggage racks on hearses, right?"

Other people don't always share my dad's outlook. In fact, some of the most contentious arguments among surviving family members can be concerned with "who gets what and why." If your elder has concerns about this subject and wants your family to avoid these kinds of recriminations, have him make a list of those objects he wants to be sure will have a good "home." In fact, have him explain the thinking in writing and attach it to a legacy letter.

For what to do with the rest of your elder's earthly treasures, consider meditating on my father's philosophy and those of the great spiritual teachers over the course of time. There is much that will leave our sphere of control when we take our last breath, and that applies in an immediate sense to our stuff. We really don't take anything material with us, and what's most important about what we leave behind cannot be quantified.

If you'd like to read more on this subject—and receive some practical advice—check out the following resources:

Blessed by Less: Clearing Your Life of Clutter by Living Lightly by Susan V. Vogt

Falling Upward: A Spirituality for the Two Halves of Life by Richard Rohr, OFM

The Force of Character and the Lasting Life by James Hillman

The Great Chain of Being: Simplifying Our Lives (Order MP3 at http://store. cac.org/Great-Chain-of-Being-Simplifying-Our-Lives-MP3_p_222.html)

How to Simplify Your Life: Seven Practical Steps to Letting Go of Your Burdens and Living a Happier Life by Werner Tiki Kustenmacher and Lothar Seiwert

Shed Your Stuff, Change Your Life: A Four-Step Guide to Getting Unstuck by Julie Morgenstern

THREE QUESTION CLUSTERS TO HELP WITH MAKING PHILOSOPHICALLY AND SPIRITUALLY INFORMED DECISIONS

In his book, *Being Mortal: Medicine and What Matters in the End*, Dr. Atul Gawande writes, "For all but our most recent history, death was a common, ever-present possibility. It didn't matter if you were five or fifty. Every day was a roll of the dice. . . . Life and death would putter on nicely, not a problem in the world. Then illness would hit and the bottom would drop out like a trap door."[3] In other words, until very recently, medical professionals had a limited range of options with which to cure serious illness or even to slow its lethal advance. When people got sick with cancer or any of the host of diseases that compromised their lungs, heart, or other vital organs, their decline and death came quickly.

Today, however, modern medical advances have made possible the cure of many serious illnesses or have, at least, stalled their unrelenting progress toward a patient's death. As Richard Groves and Henriette Klauser point out in their book, *The American Book of Dying: Lessons in Healing Spiritual Pain*, 80 percent of Americans die in bed. "The majority of us will die a natural death due to long-term disease or the aging process. . . . That means we are far more likely than our ancestors to have ample time to prepare for our own death and the deaths of those we love."[4] That also means that, as opposed to our ancestors, many of us will have a lot more time to do our spiritual work of reflecting upon the meaning and purpose of our lives.

Unfortunately, however, we can often spend these extra weeks, months—and perhaps years—in pursuit of a cure that is not forthcoming, which means that, as one physician remarked, "patients die sicker than they used to." Chemotherapy, radiation, surgery, and other treatments for life-threatening illness can prolong life—but they also can prolong and complicate the dying process as well.

Increasingly, wisdom suggests that, along with decisions regarding treatments, patients and families living with terminal illness should ask themselves and their care providers at each juncture, "What time is it?"[5] That is, given the subjective data of a patient's age, overall health, chance of recovery or at least remission, is it time to change the focus of care from attempting to overcome the illness to managing its symptoms? This is a complex question that is unique to each person and family. But there are three "question clusters" that, when considered seriously, can help patients and families make philosophically and spiritually informed decisions:

1. What is my medical condition? Have the procedures I've undergone had the desired effect, or at least been successful enough to continue? What do my medical care providers see as my "best case" scenario? What does my ideal death look like and what systems can be put in place to accomplish that end?
2. What are the most important goals I have at this point in my life? What "work" do I have left to do? Are there projects I want to complete, places I want to see, damaged relationships I want to heal? Do I have vocational goals I still want to achieve? What are my spiritual needs?
3. Given what's most important to me at this time, how will the medical procedures I'm being asked to consider help or hinder my progress in completing the goals I have set for myself?

These are questions only you can answer for yourself. But you owe it to yourself, your loved ones, and your care providers to work through them, so you can make the most of the time you have.

I suggest you consider talking through these questions with your family, your ALCM, your spiritual advisor, your physician, or a trusted friend who can serve as a good sounding board. It helps to hear yourself talking and to get the responses of concerned others.

SOURCES TO HELP WITH HARD CHOICES

Forms

Advance Directive: An advance directive is a legal document that details how you want to be treated at the end of your life if you cannot express your wishes at that time. It can contain numerous directions including such subjects as artificial nutrition and hydration, guidelines on intubation and ventilator placement—in short, what you would want to say if you could. As part of an advance directive, you can appoint an HCPOA, a person to speak for you if you cannot speak for yourself. That individual will be empowered to make choices for your care in those circumstances that are not covered in your advance directive. Obviously, you will want to be confident the person you appoint shares your values and agrees to abide by them in a critical situation. Advance directive forms are readily available through elder law attorneys, physicians, etc. You also can download your state's advance directive by visiting http://www.caringinfo.org.

POLST: If you are physically frail, have a serious medical condition, or have a life-threatening illness, talk with your physician or other medical care provider about filling out a POLST form. A POLST is a doctor's order describing in detail how you want to be cared for in the event of a life-threatening situation such as cardiac arrest. It allows for a wide range of treatments, from full resuscitation to comfort measures only. Completing a POLST form gives you say over how you are treated and relieves your family of the responsibility—and the attendant emotional, moral, and spiritual burden—of making decisions at a critical time when any decision they might have to make is fraught with ambiguity. Check out http://www.polst.org and refer to the section of this book that addresses legal issues.

Online Information

- **National Hospice and Palliative Care Organization:** The National Hospice and Palliative Care Organization (NHPCO) has published "Caring Connections," a web page that provides insightful end-of-life information. Visit http://www.nhpco.org/learn-about-end-life-care.
- **Family Caregiver Alliance:** This organization has a web page that summarizes the dynamics and decisions surrounding end-of-life care. Visit https://caregiver.org/end-life-decision-making.

Videos

- **Dr. Ira Byock on "Saying the Four Things That Matter Most for Living and Dying Well":** This video captures renowned U.S. palliative care physician and author Dr. Ira Byock making a presentation during National Palliative Care Week 2013 in Melbourne, Australia; https://www.youtube.com/watch?v=EcEQsQyYaEk.
- **Dr. Ira Byock on "The Best Care Possible through the End of Life: What It Is and How to Get It":** This video captures Dr. Byock speak-

ing in Portland, Oregon, on January 25, 2013; https://www.youtube.com/watch?v=dfxC9Km7x6Q.
- **Dr. Ira Byock on "Mortality, Morality, and the Meaning of Life":** Dr. Byock gave this speech in Eugene, Oregon, on January 24, 2013; https://www.youtube.com/watch?v=bdMKT6VJBdI.
- **Dr. Atul Gawande on "How Do We Heal Medicine?"** Dr. Gawande discusses how to deal with the difficulties encountered by modern medical practices; https://www.youtube.com/watch?v=L3QkaS249Bc.
- **West Virginia Public Broadcasting's: "The Last Chapter—End of Life Decisions":** This one-hour program examines end-of-life care options and the need for advance directives. The show focuses on empowering individuals to have the last word on how they live at the end of their lives; https://www.youtube.com/watch?v=8jKUZ8lS9b4.

HOSPICE: HELP AND HOPE IN A HARD TIME

Since its beginnings in eleventh-century Europe, hospice care has focused on five areas of comfort for persons living with terminal illness:

- Physical
- Psychological
- Social
- Spiritual
- Practical

Under the "umbrella" of hospice, an interdisciplinary team of healthcare professionals addresses a patient's care once a physician deems that patient has less than six months to live. Whereas you can find more information about hospice enrollment and what's offered by hospice care programs in the "Medical" section of this book, we want to focus herein on the spiritual dimensions of good hospice care. As a starter, consider what's going on in your life from four perspectives, expressed in "question clusters":[6]

1. **Strength:** During this time of your life, what is the source of your *strength*? What gives you the fortitude you need to face each day? Where do you go to get it?
2. **Security:** What is the source of your *security*? What makes you feel safe when events threaten to overwhelm you? Where do you find it?
3. **Peace:** What is the source of your *peace*? Where do you find equilibrium at a time of imbalance and uncertainty?

4. **Hope:** What is the source of your *hope*? Actually, what does "hope" mean to you? Is hope essentially a wish that you will be restored to perfect health or, at least, to the condition that you were in before you got sick? Is it something more? Does your sense of hope call to you from the defined past or does it beckon you forward toward an unrealized future?

Now consider how your answers to these four question clusters impact your ability to live through the days of your illness. Is there something else for which you are waiting? What might that be, and how can your caregivers help you seek it out? As you reflect upon these ideas, you may want to write in your journal or refer back to the journal entries you made when you created your legacy letter.

HOW TO BE (NOT DO) WITH DYING

In his essay "Born Toward Dying," the late Fr. Richard John Neuhaus wrote, "It used to be that we accompanied sisters and brothers to their final encounter. Now we mostly sit by and wait. The last moment that we are really with them, and they with us, is often hours or even many days before they die."[7] There are reasons for this, of course. As was noted earlier, given the advances of modern medical technology, people often die sicker than they used to. That means that controlling their pain may require stronger and more-sedating medication than might have been necessary earlier in the disease progress.

A daughter was sitting at the bedside of her comatose mother as her mother was living through the last moments of life. In the final hours, the mother's breaths decreased in strength, and the time between them increased to the point where each exhalation seemed certainly to be the last. But it wasn't. Indeed, the daughter felt that, with each exhalation, she was being brought with her mother to the great precipice where the descent into her mother's death was certain, only to be pulled back at the last possible moment by an impossibly deep gulp of air. She said to the chaplain sitting next to her, "This waiting is killing me."

Kairos Time

Most of us think of waiting in chronological terms; we wait for the bus to come, for the concert to start, for a long, sleepless night to end at dawn. This was certainly how this daughter understood her vigil. She was, in fact, waiting for her mother to die, wondering what time of the day or night that might happen. So the chaplain asked her to consider that keeping vigil at her mother's bedside was of a different sort. It wasn't chronological, or clock, time; rather, it was best defined by a Greek word: *Kairos*.

The Merriam-Webster dictionary defines *Kairos* time as that time "when conditions are right for the accomplishment of a crucial action." In this case, her mother's death was the "crucial action" for which her daughter was waiting. When she opened herself to this understanding, the daughter saw that her "waiting" could be an acceptance of what the present moment was bringing: the end of breath or another breath. She let go of her grasping and her tension so that she could truly be with her mother on the last steps of their journey as they waited together for the "right" time.

Hospice professionals and seasoned volunteers report that how one sits with a dying person will have a strong influence on the dying person's emotional state. If there is antagonism or outright hostility among family members gathered at the bedside of a dying relative, that may well be reflected in the person's agitated gestures and facial expressions. In the same way, if family members are overcome with grief and projecting a longing that the person not die, that also can complicate and prolong the dying process.

So How to Be?

- **Allow a healthy self-centeredness.** The first requirement for the empathic and caring accompaniment of a dying person is a *healthy self-centeredness*. The ancient kabbalistic tradition of *tsimtsum* teaches that, "I must withdraw to make room for the other."[8] In the present case, I can't fill up the room with *my* emotions, *my* needs, or *my* ideas. Rather, I must withdraw all my biases, my judgments, and my ego in order for the awareness of the dying person to have room to expand and grow in these final moments.
- **Have a compassionate detachment.** As Ram Dass teaches, I must ask myself in each moment, before and while giving any care, "Who is helping and who is being helped?" In a phrase, I must have as my personal goal a *compassionate detachment* from my actions, so that I do what I do with the right intention, free at any moment to change course or to stop doing or saying anything that doesn't seem helpful.
- **Ensure a clutter-free space.** It should go without saying that the space around the dying person should be free of all kinds of clutter—physical as well as emotional—or relational "junk." This is why dying at home or at least in a facility established to support the dying process is preferred. But if a loved one is in a hospital or other medical environment, strive to

create as quiet and open a space as possible. Ask staff to refrain from any tasks other than those necessary to give comfort. Turn down lights. Turn off electrical devices (including phones). Ask staff to keep overhead announcements or pages to a minimum.

- **Take cues from the dying person.** Some people may feel at home with the sound of conversation and the activities of daily life, as well as all kinds of music. An elderly woman was asked if she would like to hear any music. She replied, "Yes. I like old-time Gospel music—and Led Zeppelin." She died just after the closing strains of "Stairway to Heaven" faded into the silence of her room. But it's also true that more than one patient has asked for the harpist to leave the room because the sound irritated her. It's to the credit of harpists that they don't take it personally but, rather, understand that each person dies in her own way.
- **Ask the "WAIT" question.** Most all who teach the care of the dying counsel speaking softly and slowly words of encouragement, prayers appropriate to the dying person's spiritual orientation, and assurances that surviving loved ones will be all right. All these instructions are valid, but an admonition is also in order. Staying close to the person, being open to whatever messages I receive from my observations and intuitions in the moment, may cause me to ask the "WAIT" question: Why Am I Talking?[9] One also could include other therapeutic interventions designed to facilitate a peaceful death: Why Am I Playing Music? Why Am I Singing? Why Am I Reading? If I cannot honestly judge that my concern is for the dying one and not for myself, I need to stop.

For more tips on vigiling and establishing sacred presence at the end of life, check out the work of the **Sacred Dying Foundation** at http://www.sacred dying.org.

DEALING WITH THE DEAD

As noted in the introduction, many people in contemporary American culture seem to understand death as an accident, the result of medical malpractice, or just bad luck—for someone else. Contemplating the reality of one's own limited life span is not a popular practice in our time. But it is in the very meditation on our own mortality and the acceptance of it that the opportunity lies to make good choices about how we want to be treated in the days leading up to and following our own death.

This section will discuss the decisions you will need to make (or someone will have to make on your behalf) at the end of your life. Those decisions will reflect the meaning and the ends to which you have given to your life and the legacy you wish to leave behind.

THE BODY

Let's begin with some foundational principles with which to "ground" our discussion. In *The Good Funeral*, a book which he coauthored with Thomas Long, Thomas Lynch writes: "(H)ow we deal with our dead in their physical reality and how we deal with death as an existential reality define and describe us in primary ways. . . Ours is the species that deals with death (the idea of the thing) by dealing with our dead (the physical fact of the thing itself)."[10]

Essentially, death—our death or the death of any human being, for that matter—presents us with a problem. A body once animated by life force is no longer a living, breathing being, but what remains of the person we knew. And that body, though no longer identified by the personality that animated it, will continue to change in ways that call attention to its new reality. As survivors, we have to deal with that reality, and how we do that will depend on the meaning we attach to the body and what we do with it.

There are essentially three ways to deal with a dead body: We can bury it, entomb it, or burn it, with or without ceremony or minimal preparation. Let's look at these options in order:

- **Earth Burial.** Bodies can be buried in a casket, with or without any special preparation in most cases. "Natural" burial, in which the unembalmed body is buried directly in the ground or in a biodegradable container or shroud, also has become an increasingly attractive option for some. In some religious traditions, the body is an integral part of the leave-taking ritual and so may be present at a service and buried afterward. In others—and according to preference—the body may be buried directly with or without a service following.
- **Entombment.** In this scenario, the body is embalmed and placed in a casket, which is then placed in an above-ground vault in a building called a mausoleum.
- **Cremation.** In this process, bodies are placed in a crematory (called a "retort") and subjected to a highly heated gas fire, which burns away everything that isn't bone material or metal. Afterward, the bone fragments are recovered and run through a pulverizing machine that reduces them to a fine, white powdery dust, sometimes mistakenly referred to as ashes. The remains can then be buried, scattered, or placed in an urn. This urn can then

be placed in any number of sites, from a niche in a columbarium to a special place in a survivor's home. (This is not as uncommon as you might think.)

For further details on each of these options, please consult the "Funeral Planning Resources" page at the end of this section.

FUNERAL PLANNING: WHAT MAKES FOR A GOOD "GOOD-BYE"?[11]

Note: You may have decided that, based on your personal preferences, you don't want to have any kind of memorial service or celebration of life—any organized event. If that's the case, then the following information may not be directly relevant to you. We urge you, nonetheless, to read through it anyway, if only to understand the possible motivations behind a different approach.

In his elegy written for the Irish poet W. B. Yeats, W. H. Auden wrote of his deceased friend: "He has become his admirers," a stylistic way of saying that, after one dies, one's life is subject to the interpretation of her or his survivors. With this in mind, we'd like to take this opportunity to remind you that your leave-taking ritual is your final chance to tell people you care about and who care about you just who you were, what motivated you, and what gave ultimate meaning to you in your life. It's an opportunity to communicate your truth, which is much more than just a listing of facts (where you lived, what you did for a living, and so on). So what makes for a good "good-bye?" Consider addressing these three major functions of leave-taking rituals:

1. **To Acknowledge a Loved One Has Died.** How do you want communicated to others that you have died? How will your leave-taking ritual tell people that, yes, you're dead? This is not the place to debate the relative merits of viewings or having your body or cremated remains present at a memorial, but you will want to consider your feelings about this issue. In earlier times, the traditions of the family, religious group, or civil community dictated the process. When a person died, he or she was often washed, dressed, and laid out in the home. People were invited to come and sit with the dead person as a way of honoring him or her and absorbing the enormity of a change in the relationship. This is sometimes called a *wake*, which refers to "staying awake" to keep vigil with the deceased. In today's world, if you have a particular religious affiliation, you may want to be guided by the traditions of that organization. To that end, you will seek the advice of your group leadership. However, you also may choose to plan

your own service. There are a number of resources available for this work, as noted under "Funeral Planning Resources" at the end of this section.

2. **To Remember and Celebrate the Deceased Person's Life within the Context of His or Her Ultimate Commitments.** For many people today, the funeral or memorial service is the only part of the three-part leave-taking process that is well attended. But, to paraphrase the words of poet and funeral director Thomas Lynch, it's common today that the only one *not* invited to the funeral is the dead person.[12] As noted previously, a memorial or funeral is your final opportunity to communicate what defined your life in this dimension and what your hopes might be for those who survive you. Although the service may well contain a retrospective of your experiences, it also can be an exploration of what lay behind the choices you made and the events that shaped you.

3. **To Commend the Person to Whatever Comes Next.** The commendation of the deceased is often associated with the final surrender of one's earthly remains: to the ground, to the water—perhaps to the air. This part of your leave-taking may be connected to a particular ritual: a prayer, a blessing, a poem, a time of reverent silence, or perhaps simply the act of burial or interment. In any case, it makes the point that your life has come to a close and the relationship with those you love has been irrevocably changed. In other words, it marks the beginning, not the end, of a time of moving into a new relationship with the deceased and finding an emotional and spiritual place for him in the patchwork quilt of your life.

No matter how you do these three steps—in an orderly, liturgical process over days or in a short, spare ceremony—you will want to decide how you want others to walk through them for you.

PRAGMATIC PRACTICE: A DECISION GUIDE

Many organizations offer forms to fill out so you can detail your wishes about what happens to your body after death and what sort of memorial service you will have. For example, see **"After-Death Planning Form"** at http://www.galenpress.com/extras/adp.pdf or the **Duke Human Resources/MetLife "Funeral Planning Guide"** at http://www.hr.duke.edu/benefits/finance/life/Funeral%20Planning%20Guide.pdf.

Optimally, you will make some choices and then discuss them with your relatives or whomever will make your funeral arrangements. The information will assure your survivors they have done what you wanted. It also will help them to avoid the pressure of casket, cemetery, and funeral salespeople.

Because this information needs to be immediately available upon death, do not keep this checklist in a safe deposit box, where it might take days or weeks to discover. Instead, write out the answers to these basic questions or go to https://rowman.com/ISBN/9781442265462 to print the "After-Life Decision Guide." Once you fill out the guide or the forms noted previously, then print out copies of your responses, share them with your family, and store them in an obvious place.

We warmly acknowledge that making decisions about what happens to your body after death is emotionally challenging. We only hope that completing the process will allow you to feel confident that your truths and wishes will be carried out after your passing.

Immediately upon Death

Are there postmortem rituals you would like to have observed? For example, would you like your body to be washed by a loved one? Would you like to be dressed in certain clothing? Do you want to be wrapped in a special quilt?

What Do You Want Your Survivors to Do with Your Earthly Remains?

- Earth burial. Where?
  - In a coffin. Do you have one picked out or purchased? If so, from where?
  - If not, do you have a preference for the type of coffin, and, if yes, what would you like?
  - Directly into the ground ("natural" burial). Where? If you already own a burial plot, where is it? Name of cemetery/mausoleum? Phone number? Location/plot number? Location of your contract?
- Burial at sea.
  - Cremation with burial. Burial where?
  - If burial, do you have a vessel picked out or purchased? If so, from where?
  - If not, do you have a preference for the type of vessel, and, if yes, what would you like?
- Cremation with scattering. Scattering where?

Whether you choose burial or cremation, be aware of what happens if you die away from home. How does your body get from the funeral home or crematorium? How much will the transportation cost? If you have made arrangements to be cremated in your hometown and die abroad, your body will have to be transported in a coffin to your hometown unless you purchase particular "packages" and insurance. For details on this dilemma, contact your local crematorium.

Also, for information on legal and ethical considerations on scattering ashes, visit: http://www.cremationsolutions.com/Scattering-Ashes-Laws-Regulations-c108.html. The website provides an overview of state and federal regulations regarding the scattering of cremated remains.

Who's Going to Do This Work?

Do you need the services of a funeral director? If yes, has your family been served well in the past by someone or a particular company that you would choose to coordinate your burial? If yes, who is it? Funeral home name? Person to contact? Phone number?

Are you seeking a direct cremation? If yes, do you know the crematorium you would like your survivors to contact upon your death? If yes, who is it? Crematorium name? Person to contact? Phone number?

When choosing your funeral home or crematorium, is price a consideration? Charges can vary widely. Remember, after-death care is a service for which we pay, just as we pay our other bills. Seeking the best overall price, service, and quality does not dishonor your loved one, nor does it necessarily reflect your love for the person.

Do you need the services of a religious leader? If yes, who would you like your survivors to contact? Religious leader? Worship community? Phone number?

When?

- Do you want to be buried or have your ashes spread or buried within a certain time frame? If so, when?
- Are you a member of a religious community that specifies time limitations on cremation or burial?

What Type of Celebration of Life Do You Envision?

Traditional funeral? Celebration of life? Wake? Vigil? Viewing?

Where?

- If you would like to have a funeral or memorial service, where would you like it to be held?
- Are you looking for a funeral home that has a nice chapel or room for an event? If yes, note any requests or suggestions of places to contact.

- Or are you a member of a worship community or other organization that can or will hold your funeral or memorial service? If yes, what is it? Who is the contact?

Details to Consider

- Is it important to you that your body be present at your memorial service?
- What sacred rituals would you like to commemorate your passing—and who will do them (e.g., sitting shiva, burning a candle for seven days, having a church choir sing, releasing doves or balloons, having pallbearers carry the casket [who would you like to be asked?], having a group say the rosary, being wrapped in a quilt shroud)?
- If you have a religious service, is there a traditional format you want followed or would you prefer only certain elements be included?
- Are there cultural or heritage traditions you want to include in the memorial service?
- Did you serve in the military? If yes, which branch? If yes, would you like to have a flag ceremony as part of your memorial service?
- What music, if any, do you want played and how (e.g., organ, flute, harp)?
- Are there particular prayers, readings, or poems you would like to have read and by whom?
- Who would you like to attend or to be notified?
- If friends and family want to honor you with memorial contributions, what are your wishes? Do you want flowers? Masses said in your memory? Do you have special charities to which you would encourage them to contribute? If yes, what are they?

Planning a Celebration of Life Event

Some people want their families and friends to experience a joyful celebration of life with good food and drink, stories being shared, maybe even dancing.

- Would you like this type of event? If yes, *when* should it take place? Immediately after your funeral or memorial service? At a later date? At the convenience of your family and friends?
- Do you have a *place* in mind for this event (Favorite restaurant? Church hall? Temple lobby? Ballroom?)?
- *Who* would you like to attend?
- Is there any *particular food* you want at your event? If so, what kind? Do any foods have special meaning to you? Share your story.
- What *special elements* should be incorporated into your celebration of life party? For example: Do you have favorite colors? Do you want certain

treasures or photos displayed? Do you want a guest book, prayer cards, or memorial cards? Do you want time set aside for people to speak? Do you want special music played? Do you want your family and friends to play games and dance? Do you want stories or poems read? If so, by whom?

- Is there someone you would like to have as the "master of ceremonies" for the event? If yes, who?
- Do you want to record a *video of you sharing your life legacy* or create a slide presentation with music and captions to share your life? Or, do you want someone to do this for you?
- Do you have *pets*? Would you like them to be included? If so, how?

Now take a few moments and close your eyes. Imagine this special celebration of You. Walk through the event in your mind and notice who is there and what it sounds like. Are there special smells? Does it look the way you have planned? Consider all the elements, and then see how that feels to you. Does it achieve what you want? Is it simple enough? Is it loud enough? Does it convey your sacred wish? Does it honor your legacy? Now go back through your plan and make any changes you considered.

> For downloadable forms to use in **"Planning a Celebration of Life"** and for **"Writing My Own Obituary,"** go to https://rowman.com/ISBN/978144 2265462.

MY WAY: WRITING YOUR OWN OBITUARY

As noted earlier, one important element in a leave-taking ritual is a remembrance and celebration of the deceased person's life within the context of his or her ultimate commitments. This guideline applies to a person's obituary as well. A good obituary is much more than a list of dates and activities: It's a retrospective of a life with a thematic center. As such, it requires some reflection.

Your elder might be interested in writing his or her own obituary. If that's the case, have him ponder these guidelines:

- As you think about what you've done in your life, take some time to think about why. For example, if you enjoyed fishing, you might want to reflect on what about it appealed to you. Was it the opportunity to be out in nature, or was it perhaps an activity you could share with your family?
- What motivated you to persevere when your work or some other important part of your life became difficult?

- As you reflect on your life, what accomplishment has given you the greatest satisfaction and why?
- No matter how much space is allotted for an obituary, try to give your reader a sense of what gave your life meaning. You might even want to jot down ideas and begin drafting your final words to the world.

Practical Considerations, or How Much Is Your Story Worth?

For the most part, the days of free obituary notices are gone; and, quite frankly, for a long time there was not much more to them than one's name, family dates of birth and death, and time of funeral or memorial service—if that. Now, obituaries published in newspapers can be very expensive. For example, my local newspaper charges $100 per column inch.

There are many less-expensive alternatives, particularly for users of the Internet and social media. As part of the funeral package you purchase, your after-death care provider may furnish a low- or no-cost web page where family members can post obituary and service information. If your provider doesn't offer this option, you might want to check out the following websites:

- http://memorialwebsites.legacy.com/
- http://memorial.yourtribute.com/pricing.aspx
- http://www.christianmemorials.com/

If you have a blog or if most of the people you want to notify are Facebook "friends," you can post an obituary there. You also can create a temporary Facebook page just for that purpose. Can you post a 140-character link to your own blog or Facebook page on Twitter? You can double the potential reach of your notice.

Additional Resources on Obituaries

https://www.caring.com/articles/placing-an-obituary
http://www.nolo.com/legal-encyclopedia/how-write-obituary.html
http://www.imsorrytohear.com/blog/obituaries-and-death-notices-explained
For instructions on posting an obituary on WordPress, go to http://www.
   screencast.com/t/c1wNRK3Is.

SPECIAL CONSIDERATIONS FOR THE LGBT COMMUNITY

Whether we are willing to admit it or not, some segments of society are still not open and welcoming to our LGBT brothers and sisters. One way to ensure that you are honored and remembered in the way you would like to be is to be forthright regarding to what extent and in what manner you want your sexual orientation to be disclosed and discussed.

> For a **special form for LGBT elders** to fill out that would highlight their after-life wishes regarding their sexual orientation and partner, go to https://rowman.com/ISBN/9781442265462.

After filling out the form, it would be prudent to be sure the form is kept with other important documents.

Also, if you are living in what you consider a permanent committed relationship, be sure to seek out competent legal advice regarding your mutual rights as a couple and do what you need to do to ensure you are recognized as a couple in your state. More than one couple has discovered—at the worst possible time—that each partner had no legal standing with regard to the other's assets, medical affairs, or after-death care. Take the time to complete the necessary legal paperwork!

For more information on this subject, visit these two online resources:

https://www.legalzoom.com/articles/domestic-partnership-vs-marriage-the-legal-advantages-and-disadvantages-of-each

http://www.glad.org/uploads/docs/publications/legal-planning-couples.pdf

FUNERAL PLANNING RESOURCES

Funeral Consumers Alliance: This organization offers a comprehensive website filled with information about options for after-death care including home-based funerals; http://funerals.org.

Religious Sources/Checklists and Short Publications

Caution: Regardless of what the larger tradition in any religious community prescribes, individuals and families invariably adopt—and often adapt—those practices which bring them healing. It's important not to assume that an individual or a family will follow all or any of the conventions of the wider group.

General Reference:
- *Death and Bereavement Across Cultures*, by Colin Murray Parkes, Pittu Laungani, and William Young, editors (1997)
- *Death and Dying in World Religions*, by Lucy Bregman, editor (2009)
- *The Sacred Art of Dying: How World Religions Understand Death*, by Kenneth Kramer (1988)

Buddhist:
- *Death and Dying in the Tibetan Buddhist Tradition*, compiled by Ven. Pende Hawter; http://www.buddhanet.net/deathtib.htm
- *The Tibetan Book of Living and Dying*, Revised and Updated Version, by Sogyal Rinpoche (2002)

Christian:
- Everplans: An online guide to the after-death practices of a number of Christian communities; https://www.everplans.com/articles/christian-funeral-traditions
- *Now and at the Hour of Our Death: Instructions Concerning My Death and Funeral*, Revised Edition, by Peter Gilmour and David A. Lysik (Liturgy Training Publications, 1999, ISBN 978-1-56854-286-7). This short booklet, published by the Roman Catholic Archdiocese of Chicago, can be very useful for Roman Catholics and others in the wider Catholic tradition. There are places throughout the booklet to list important information as well as your own choices for your service.

Hindu:
- *Religion, Death and Dying,* ed. by Lucy Bregman. Vol. 3, Chapter 7 (2009)
- "Grieving Tradition in a New Land: Hindu Death and Dying Rituals in America," by Kyoko Murata; http://www2.gsu.edu/~wwwrel/Grieving_Tradition_in_a_New_Land.pdf

Islamic:
- "Funeral Rites in Islam: Everyone Shall Taste Death." A web page offering a concise overview of Islamic after-death practices; http://www.islamreligion.com/articles/4946/viewall
- *Authentic Step-by-Step Illustrated Janazah Guide,* by Mohamed Ebrahim Siala. Explains Muslim practices for the care of the dead; http://www.missionislam.com/knowledge/janazahstepbystep.htm

Jewish:
- *The Jewish Way in Death and Mourning*, by Maurice Lamm. A comprehensive overview of Jewish practices regarding death, burial and bereavement; http://www.chabad.org/library/article_cdo/aid/281541/jewish/The-Jewish-Way-in-Death-and-Mourning.htm

TRADITIONAL PRAYERS FOR THE DEAD

Anglican Prayer for the Dead

O God, whose mercies cannot be numbered: Accept our
prayers on behalf of thy servant N., and grant him an
entrance into the land of light and joy, in the fellowship of

thy saints; through Jesus Christ thy Son our Lord, who liveth
and reigneth with thee and the Holy Spirit, on God, now
and forever. Amen.

Bahai Prayer for the Dead

O, my God! This is Thy servant and the son of Thy servant who hath believed in Thee
and in Thy signs, and set his face towards Thee, wholly detached from all except
Thee. Thou art, verily, of those who show mercy the most merciful.

Deal with him, O Thou Who forgivest the sins of men and concealest their faults, as
beseemeth the heaven of Thy bounty and the ocean of Thy grace. Grant him admission
within the precincts of Thy transcendent mercy that was before the foundation of earth
and heaven. There is no God but Thee, the Ever-Forgiving, the Most Generous.

Catholic Prayer for the Dead

Eternal rest grant unto him (her), O Lord, and let perpetual light shine upon him (her).
May he (she) rest in peace. Amen.

May his/her soul and the souls of all the faithful departed, through the mercy of God,
rest in peace.

Amen.

Hindu Prayer for the Dead

The wise have said that Atman is immortal: And that the phenomenon of death is
merely the separation of the astral body from the physical body. The five elements
of which the body is composed return to their source. Our scriptures teach us that as
pilgrims unite and separate at a public inn, so also fathers, mothers, sons, brothers,
wives, relations unite and separate in this world. He who thus understands the
nature of the body and all human relationships based upon it will derive strength to
bear the loss of our dear ones. In Divine plan, one day each union must end with
separation.

Jewish Prayer for the Dead: Mourner's Kaddish

Exalted and hallowed be His great Name. (Cong: "Amen.")

Throughout the world which He has created according to His Will, may He establish
His kingship, bring forth His redemption and hasten the coming of His Moshiach.
(Cong: "Amen.")

In your lifetime and in your days and in the lifetime of the entire House of Israel,
speedily and soon, and say, Amen.

(Cong: "Amen. May His great Name be blessed forever and to all eternity, blessed.")

May His great Name be blessed forever and to all eternity. Blessed and praised,
glorified, exalted and extolled, honored, adored and lauded be the Name of the
Holy One, blessed be He. (Cong: "Amen.")

Beyond all the blessings, hymns, praises and consolations that are uttered in the
world; and say, Amen. (Cong: "Amen.")
May there be abundant peace from heaven, and a good life for us and for all Israel;
and say, Amen. (Cong: "Amen.")
He Who makes peace in His heavens, may He make peace for us and for all Israel;
and say, Amen. (Cong: "Amen.")

Muslim Prayer: Al-Fatiha

In the name of God, the Entirely Merciful, the Especially Merciful.
All praise and thanks is due to God, [The] Creator, Owner, Sustainer of the Worlds.
The Entirely Merciful, The Especially Merciful.
Owner of the Day of Recompense.
You alone do we worship and You alone we seek for help.
Guide us to the Straight Path.
The path of those whom Your blessings are upon, Not of those who You have cursed
nor of those who have gone astray.

DEATH DIALOGUE

In his popular work *The Seven Habits of Highly Effective People*, the late
writer and speaker Steven Covey wrote that, in considering any life path or
project, we need to begin "with the end in mind."[13] Our ancestors certainly
embraced that notion. In the Hebrew Scriptures, the Psalmist prays, "Teach
us to number our days aright/that we may gain wisdom of heart" (Ps. 90:12),
an admonition shared by virtually all spiritual traditions. How can we ponder
that question today, when so many of us may not have a place where we can
speak openly about our feelings and fears of death?

In this section, we'll examine a few dialogues currently going on in
America. We do so with the hope that we may inspire you to get involved in
the conversation.

BODY AND ORGAN DONATION: LOVE AND LOGISTICS

Most of us assume that death will occur after a decline that takes place
over time, usually from a debilitating disease such as cancer or heart disease—or just advanced age, for that matter. Given that assumption, we
don't think much about organ or body donation. There are age limits on
these kinds of donations, and, for the most part, we assume that we won't
be eligible, that our bodies will be pretty much "used up" by that time. Not
necessarily.

First, even if we're past the age for some kinds of donations, we can still donate some body parts for research. Second, most of us have no idea how or when we will die. People of a certain age die without prior notice every day, the only evidence of a fatal illness or condition being sudden death. And, of course, accidents can occur at any time to anyone. So it's never too late or too early to consider one's feelings about donating part or all of our body, to whom and under what conditions.

Many people have donated a kidney to someone who needed it and who matched the receiver's biological makeup. Given that the liver is the one internal organ that can regrow itself (albeit in limited ways), a portion of a liver can be taken from one person and transplanted into another. Following death, virtually all the major organs can be transplanted, assuming a healthy organ and a suitable recipient. And, of course, medical schools are almost always seeking whole body donations for education and research.

The great majority of religious traditions either offer no definitive teaching or encourage donating part or all of our body following death—and sometimes during life. Each of us will have to examine our own values and to discuss them with our families and/or spiritual advisors; most importantly, the time to have these discussions is *before* any crisis occurs. Sitting with families following the death of a loved one, I have observed the anguish of the survivors as they attempted to discern the will of the deceased and to process their own issues. The stress of this time is often compounded exponentially by the uncertainties left behind, most of which can be eliminated by talking with one another and communicating your desires *in writing*, using an advance directive and appointing a HCPOA who can speak on your behalf, as noted in the "Medical" section of this guide.

Resource for Information on Organ and Body Donation

http://organdonor.gov: Comprehensive site sponsored by the federal government with links to each of the fifty states

TO PULL OR NOT TO PULL: HOW TO ASK THE QUESTION

Eighty-five-year-old Alan lay immobile on his hospital bed, surrounded by his family, the attending physician, and the hospital chaplain. Having suffered a heart attack followed by a stroke, Alan had been intubated to help him breathe. Numerous chemicals were dripping into his body through tubes connected to sites on his chest and arms. His condition had deteriorated steadily since being admitted through the emergency department three days earlier, and now the doctor had come to his family to tell them Alan's kidneys had begun to fail. "We could start dialysis," the doctor told the family, "but I don't think it would help him at all. I believe Alan is dying."

Alan's oldest son said to his mother, Beth: "Well, if we're not going to do anything to stop Dad from dying, why do we have him hooked up to all this stuff? Why don't we just take it off and keep him comfortable until he dies?" Alan's wife of fifty-five years turned to ask the chaplain, who was standing next to her, "But if we do that, aren't we playing God?" The chaplain replied gently, "Beth, is it possible that we've been playing God ever since we intubated him?"

As we can see from this scenario, our modern medical technology has shown us that there's much that we *can* do in a medical crisis today, but many of us lack guidance in helping us decide what we *should* do. Lacking a philosophical or theological foundation on which to build a decision-making platform, we may find ourselves torn back and forth between one decision and another. This is not the place to tell you what to do; however, following are some considerations for your beloved elder to keep in mind:

1. According to medical ethics professionals—as well as many theologians—there is no ethical difference between *withholding* and *withdrawing* a medically futile treatment. However, that doesn't mean that doctors will withdraw a treatment without the consent of the patient or his or her surrogate decision makers. There may even be cases when the doctor will refuse the request of a patient or surrogate decision maker to withdraw the treatment. Therefore, good communication with one's healthcare providers is of paramount importance, particularly as we age. Unlike the earlier narrative, withdrawal of support may mean discontinuing medical interventions for a person who has terminal dementia but is not actively dying.[14] It's imperative your healthcare providers understand and will honor your wishes.
2. The previous point presumes you have taken the time to think through your understanding of what a truly human life *is* and that you have communicated your values to loved ones, medical care providers, and anyone who has decision-making authority over your health care in the event that you don't.
3. The ongoing advance of medical technology means that we have no idea about what may be coming into our lives in years to come. Revisiting your own values and taking care to be sure they are communicated regularly to your loved ones and healthcare providers is the best way to insure that your wishes will be honored.

DEATH CAFÉS

In a growing number of places in our country today, there are such events called "Death Cafés." Death Cafés were introduced by Bernard Crettaz, a

Swiss sociologist and anthropologist who wanted to stimulate conversations among ordinary people regarding their feelings about death.

The format of Death Cafés is simple. Organizers advertise the event as an opportunity to have a discussion about a subject that's often on people's minds but which they don't often speak. People are invited to come for coffee and conversation. There are different configurations, but one person usually serves as facilitator. The leader may start with a question such as "Why are you here?" As one leader related, "Those were the last words I uttered for the rest of the session."

Time is open-ended, although most Death Cafés last two to three hours. The comments of one participant at the end of her second gathering are common: "I have always been afraid of death and, therefore, have been afraid of life, not allowing myself to do much. But since I came to the last group, I have felt less afraid, freer, like I can do more in my life."[15]

Resources

To find out more about Death Cafés and learn if they are taking place in your area or how to start one, visit http://www.deathcafe.com. On the site, you'll also find more information about the origins, purposes, and logistics of the Death Café movement.

If you'd like to host a "Death Dinner," to which you can invite your friends and acquaintances to share their thoughts on death as well as to share a nice meal, visit http://deathoverdinner.org/ for more details.

Or, explore the tools available through **The Conversation Project**, which is dedicated to helping people talk about their wishes for end-of-life care. At http://theconversationproject.org, you can, for example, order a "Conversation Starter Kit" that includes tools and tips to help you have "the conversation."

DOING IT YOURSELF:
DECIDING ON DEATH "WITH DIGNITY"

To some minds, it is an irony that, at a time in the history of medical practice when doctors can do more than ever before to alleviate the pain and other symptoms associated with terminal illness, a number of physicians and other healthcare providers—as well as political leaders and members of the public—are promoting laws that permit doctors to prescribe medications which, if taken according to the directions on the container, will result in the death of the patient. On the other hand, it's also true that, due to the advances in pharmacology and other medical technologies, the life of a terminally ill patient can be prolonged much longer than at any time up to the present—which may well mean that, as an oncologist once remarked, "People will die sicker than they used to." For example, a person with lung cancer may, with the help of modern antibiotics, be able to overcome an opportunistic pneumonia infection, the cancer will continue ravaging the lungs or even metastasize and attack the bones or other parts of the body, making the management of pain or shortness of breath much more difficult. At that point, the patient may have to choose between constant pain and severely diminished consciousness, not to mention a whole host of other problems including, but not limited to, incontinence, delirium, and the loss of any kind of independence in daily activities. Faced with the specter of a life that seems only marginally human, a logical person might conclude that the only sensible action is to end one's life.

Of course, it's not quite that simple to do—at least legally. As of 2015, only Oregon, Washington, and Vermont permit a doctor to write a lethal prescription—and then only following a complicated procedure involving multiple physicians, including a psychiatrist in some cases. Interestingly, between 1997 and January 2014, about 36 percent of "death with dignity" filled prescriptions were not used,[16] leading some observers to suggest that possessing the prescription gave patients a sense of control, a comforting factor for people who feared they might have to endure an agonizing death.

It's not the purpose of this book to argue for or against the Death with Dignity law. However, it's worth noting that patients living with terminal illness do have a choice in how they want to be treated. Patients are not obliged, nor can they be compelled, to pursue every available means to prolong their lives—or their dying—no matter how unlikely a cure or remission may be. Indeed, more than one person who, upon receiving a terminal diagnosis, has opted not to pursue aggressive therapies, choosing instead to use his remaining days to enjoy his time with loved ones, pursue a deeper spiritual life, or engage in long-postponed activities such as travel or study. Many of these people enroll in hospice as early as possible where, as noted earlier, the focus is totally on comfort.

In the end, we have the right and the responsibility to take ownership of our health care—and how we will be treated at every stage of our life. Just what that care will be and how it will be delivered should be the result of our own discernment in conversation with healthcare providers, spiritual advisors, and loved ones. The tools are available. We need to learn what they are, how they can be used, and then determine how *we* wish to use them.

For Further Exploration

To get a glimpse at how some medical providers deal with their own terminal diseases, visit "How Doctors Die: Showing Others the Way" (http://www.ny times.com/2013/11/20/your-money/how-doctors-die.html?pagewanted=all&_

r=0) and "A Fascinating Look at How Doctors Choose to Die" (http://www
.rd.com/health/healthcare/how-doctors-choose-to-die).

THE REST IS . . . SPIRITUAL PRACTICES AND POEMS

"It is the Silence which holds us all, always; / The Silence from which we come, / And the Silence to which we return."[17] To paraphrase these words of my dear friend and poet John Rose, it is from the Silence that we emerge at birth and to the Silence we return when we die. In between the two bookends of our lives are millions of words and images—a virtual onslaught of stimuli coming at us each second of our existence. Perhaps that's why the great sages and seers across the spiritual and philosophical spectrum counsel spending a significant portion of time in silence each day as a way of staying grounded in the storm of phenomena that assault our senses.

In that spirit, we end this section—and our time together—with a few contemplative practices and reflections that touch on the theme of life's end and ends. Read each selection slowly, then pause in silence and let the silence lead you to where the questions and the answers revolve around each other in an ever-expanding circle and draw you back to the place of wisdom where you began. And be well on your Journey.

Creating a Spiritual Moment with an App? App-solutely!

You will find numerous meditation practices are available for your smartphone. Check out **"3 Minute Retreat," "Calm," "Finger Labyrinth,"** and **"Inspirational Wisdom Quotes"** or search the app store for words such as mindfulness, meditation, spirituality, zen, prayer, labyrinth walking, chanting, bible, psalms, palliative care, and hospice care.

SPIRITUAL DIRECTION

"Spiritual direction" is a form of Holy listening; the Irish call it Anam Cara (Soul Friend). This practice is typically done on a monthly basis in fifty-minute sessions with a trained spiritual director. It is not pastoral care or psychotherapy. There's no "fixing" or judgment attitudes, only companioning while taking a long, loving look at the real. It is a place to listen to how the spirit is moving throughout your daily life. The Spirit is represented by the "third chair."

Spiritual direction is for anyone, but, as a practice for caregivers and elders, spiritual direction offers spiritual expansion for nurturing your self-care and wellbeing. It provides the structure for gentle, warm companioning during your caregiving journey, during an elder's aging transitions and end of life, and for grief comfort.

To find a spiritual director in your area, see the Spiritual Directors International database for your area at http://www.sdiworld.org. Rev. John Mabry, PhD, further explains how this practice works.

ABOUT SPIRITUAL DIRECTION

By Rev. John Mabry, PhD
Director, Interfaith Spiritual Direction Certificate Program
The Chaplaincy Institute
http://wwwchaplaincyinstitute.org

A lot of people who want spiritual direction do not know that such a ministry even exists. And when they find it, they often find that it does not provide easy answers as they had hoped. Instead, it focuses us on the difficult questions our lives present to us and helps us to make careful and soulful discernments, supported by a sympathetic companion.

"Spiritual direction" is a misleading description of this ministry, and yet, due to history, that is the name that most people recognize. In actuality, spiritual guides typically do not do much "directing"—particularly those using a nondirective interfaith approach. We don't tell people what to think, or what to believe, or how they are supposed to feel, or what to do in any specific circumstance.

This is good practice. What most people need is not another person—who is allegedly an "expert"—to tell them what to think or do or how to behave. A true spiritual director is good at helping people uncover that "deep down" wisdom.

If you have never been to spiritual direction, upon first glance it resembles psychotherapy. Two people sit in a room in chairs that face each other and talk for about an hour. But this is where the similarities to therapy end. In therapy you might discuss your emotional life, or perhaps why you hate your mother. In contrast, the content of the spiritual direction session is usually quite specifically focused on the seeker's spiritual life.

In spiritual direction, you might still talk about why you hate your mother, but your spiritual guide will most likely patiently wait for you to finish, and then ask you how holding on to those feelings affects your feelings of connection to the Divine. If you picture Divinity as Mother Earth, you can see how this could be very significant, indeed.

Interfaith spiritual direction is non dogmatic and noncoercive. This doesn't mean that interfaith spiritual directors are pushovers, though. People often have a difficult time with things their spiritual director has to say. This is because we in the West have typically been told that if you do A, B, and C, in the right order and without asking any inconvenient questions, your spiritual life will be dandy.

This is, of course, not the case. The spiritual journey is the most difficult thing many of us will ever endeavor to do. It means that the person we thought we were may have to die so that the person we really are can show up. It means that we may have to let go of cherished notions that no longer serve us, and that can be as difficult as prying Linus's blanket out of his fingers. And we usually don't have to do these things once, but over and over. It's excruciating, it's exhausting, and there is no road map to show us exactly how to get from here to there, and no instruction manual to tell us the "right" way to do it.

Fortunately, we don't have to do it alone. That's where spiritual direction comes in. A spiritual director will walk with you on your spiritual journey, listen as you uncover your true purpose, and support you as you discover your true path. He will point out things that you may not be able to see because they are too close to your field of vision. But you don't have to take the word of your spiritual director. You are always the expert on your spiritual life.

You also can trust your spiritual director to be truthful. A good spiritual director will not tell you only those things you want to hear. When he hears something that feels "off," he is going to bring attention to this and invite further discernment. This is good direction, and a wise person will value the director's opinion, even if he does not share it.

For many of us, spiritual direction is an essential part of our journeys. Just as you wouldn't set off across the desert alone, it helps to have a soul friend along for the journey—because when your canteen is empty, it's a good bet that your director's is not.

Spiritual directors do not have all the answers, and the good ones don't pretend to. But we do have a warm, hospitable space to offer, a cup of tea to share, and our full attention to give. It is not certainty we offer, but presence. No one needs to walk the spiritual path alone.

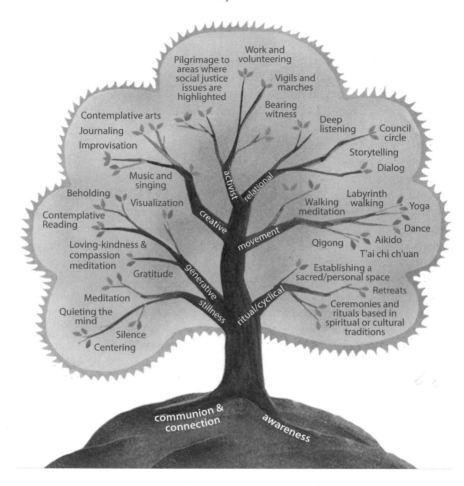

THE TREE OF CONTEMPLATIVE PRACTICES

From The Center for Contemplative Mind in Society
Concept and design by Maia Duerr
Illustration by Carrie Bergman
http://www.contemplativemind.org

The Tree illustrates some of the contemplative practices currently in use in secular organizations and academic settings. It is not intended to be comprehensive.

On the Tree of Contemplative Practices, the roots symbolize the two intentions that are the foundation of all contemplative practices: Communion/Connection and Awareness. The roots of the tree encompass and transcend differences in the religious traditions from which many of the practices originated. They also allow room for the inclusion of new practices being created in secular contexts.

The branches represent different groupings of practices. For example, *Stillness Practices* focus on quieting the mind and body in order to develop calmness and focus. *Generative Practices* may come in many different forms but share the common intent of generating thoughts and feelings, such as thoughts of devotion and compassion, rather than calming and quieting the mind. Please note that such classifications are not definitive, and many practices could be included in more than one category.

Because this illustration cannot possibly include all contemplative practices, we encourage you to create your own Tree of Contemplative Practices by downloading a blank Tree at http://www.contemplativemind.org/practices/tree and filling it in with contemplative practices you outline for yourself. Activities not included on the Tree—including those which may seem mundane, such as gardening or eating—may be understood to be contemplative practices when done with the intent of cultivating awareness and wisdom.

B.L.E.S.S. YOURSELF—5 STEPS TO MINDFUL SELF-CARE FOR CAREGIVERS

By Donald Altman, MA, LPC
Excerpted with permission from
101 Mindful Ways to Build Resilience: One-Minute Mindfulness Practices for Calm, Clarity, Optimism, and Happiness
http://www.mindfulpractices.com

Caring for others requires a lot of self-kindness, self-compassion, and self-care. Use the acronym B.L.E.S.S. to avoid burnout or compassion fatigue. Find a quiet place where you can spend three to five minutes to B.L.E.S.S. Yourself. You can do this in any position: standing, sitting, or lying down. If you are sitting in a chair, take an upright and graceful but relaxed posture. Observe a moment of silence before starting—which you can think of as a prayer or a moment for setting the intention to take care of yourself.

B—Be in the Body; Breathe

To begin, take three nice, long belly breaths as a way to get out of your busy mind and drop back into the body. The breath is your intimate kiss with this moment and wellbeing, so let your breath deepen and exhale slowly. This will help you return to center by activating your body's natural relaxation system and turning down the volume on stress and stress hormones.

L—Listen to Your Needs

Take a moment to listen inwardly. Is there a wise voice of self-care or self-compassion telling you how to take care of yourself? Open up to the message there for you. Perhaps your body is telling you to get more sleep or rest, or to take the time to eat a nutritious and mindful snack. Maybe there are emotions you feel which need to be heard. Maybe your wise self reminds you of a re-source or other help available to you. Just open and listen, without judgment, to whatever comes to you.

E—Elevate Your View

For a few moments, allow yourself to constructively distance, or elevate from, the day-to-day caregiving mode. Imagine yourself high on a hilltop looking down at all that is happening in your life and your caregiving. When caring for others, it's natural to experience the stress and feelings of uncertainty that come with loss and transition. By elevating, you shift perspective. This may allow you to see things in a fresh way and have compassion for all you are witnessing.

S—Sense and Sensitivity

Tune into and rejuvenate yourself through your senses. Get very present with your surroundings in this very moment. Listen to sounds. Look at colors—even seeing if you can find a favorite color somewhere. Notice the shapes and objects around you. Look for something pleasant you can focus on right now. Notice your feet on the floor and how rooted, secure, and grounded you are. Be sensitive to how your senses nourish you and the messages they send you, telling you when they need self-care.

S—Sacred

Acknowledge the Sacred in your caregiving. Breathe into the body as you feel a sense of the Sacred both within and surrounding you. Now, expand your gaze, letting it penetrate the beauty, preciousness, and design of all things—man-made and natural. Bask your sacred self and all around you in the warm glow of gratitude, calm, and serenity. Let yourself find the Sacred in the most ordinary work you do.

To conclude the B.L.E.S.S. Yourself practice, take a breath in as you raise both arms up above your head—like the sun rising in the sky. Now, exhale slowly as you let your arms gently come down to your sides.

THE LABYRINTH PRACTICE AS A TOOL FOR AGING WELLBEING

By Mary Jo Saavedra
Certified Labyrinth Facilitator
Adapted with permission from Veriditas
http://www.veriditas.org

Labyrinth History and Meaning

The labyrinth, an ancient pattern found in many cultures throughout the world, is a path of prayer. People throughout history have recognized and experienced its power as a walking meditation, a crucible of change, a watering hole for the spirit, and a mirror of the soul.

In essence, the practice of labyrinth walking provides an opportunity for self-discovery, innovation, and celebration as the experience integrates the body with the mind and the mind with the Spirit.

Labyrinth designs have been found on pottery, tablets, and tiles dating as far back as 5,000 years. Patterns abound; many are based on spirals and circles mirrored in nature. In Native American tradition, the labyrinth is identical to the Medicine Wheel and Man in the Maze. The Celts described the labyrinth as the Never Ending Circle. It is also known as the Kabbalah in mystical Judaism. The one feature all labyrinth designs have in common is they have one path that begins from the outer edge and winds circuitously to the center.

Currently being used worldwide as a way to quiet the mind and recover balance in life, labyrinths are open to all people as a nondenominational, cross-cultural blueprint for wellbeing where psyche meets spirit. They can be found in medical centers, parks, churches, schools, prisons, memorial parks, spas, cathedrals, and retreat centers as well as people's backyards.

How to Walk a Labyrinth

Some people come to walk a labyrinth with questions; others come just to slow down and take time out from a busy life. Some come to find strength to take a next step. Many come during times of grief and loss. Whatever the reason for showing up, a good way to begin is by sitting quietly to reflect before walking the labyrinth. Then, once grounded, take the first step.

Generally, there are three stages to a labyrinth walk: (1) Releasing on the way in, (2) receiving in the center, and (3) returning to the beginning (by taking the same path out of the labyrinth). There are no tricks to the process and no dead ends. Unlike a maze where you can lose your way, the labyrinth is a spiritual tool that can help you find your way. Symbolically, and sometimes actually, you take back out into the world that which you have received.

As there are no tricks to the process, no right way or wrong way to walk a labyrinth exists. As a caregiver, use the labyrinth any way that supports what you need (while being respectful of others walking). For example, you may go directly to the center and sit quietly or take a long time to make your way in and out. In walking with an elder, you may walk together, he may use a walker, or you may even push him in a wheelchair when the construction of the labyrinth permits.

Benefits of the Meditation Process

What labyrinth walkers find is that the Sacred is revealed through the simple rhythm of putting one foot in front of the other, turning left and then turning right, going in and coming out.

The experience transcends the limits of still meditation as both sides of the brain are activated, allowing for a holistic experience that reduces stress, quiets the mind, grounds the body, and opens the heart. In fact, several medical studies are underway to identify the impacts of labyrinth walking on dementia, brain health, and wellbeing.

Based on the circle, the universal symbol for unity and wholeness, the labyrinth enlivens the intuitive part of our nature and stirs within the human heart the longing for connectedness and the remembrance of our purpose for living. The path winds throughout and becomes a mirror for where we are in our lives; it can touch our sorrows and release our joys.—Sr. Mary Jo Chaves of the Franciscan Spiritual Center in Milwaukie, Oregon

Finding a Labyrinth in Your Area

On the Veriditas.org website, you can access a comprehensive Labyrinth Locator tool at http://labyrinthlocator.com/home. Once you input your area code, city, or country, the Locator will provide a list of public and private labyrinths in your area. It is also a wonderful tool to use when you travel, so you do not miss special experiences with labyrinths throughout the United States and abroad.

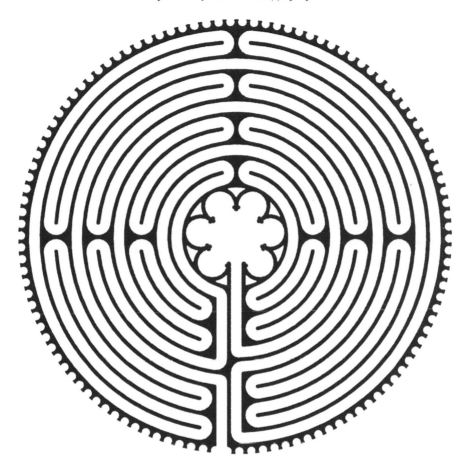

Finger and Desk Labyrinths

In addition to the walking of a labyrinth, you and your elder might enjoy a finger labyrinth for doing on the lap or a desk labyrinth for use with a stylus. Finger and desk labyrinths come in many sizes and materials. There are even double finger labyrinths that allow using both hands simultaneously, as well as labyrinth smartphone apps. These small labyrinths provide the same benefits as the walking labyrinths and are easy to use during busy caregiving, or with an elder as a wellness practice.

The labyrinth on this page is a template of the Chartres Labyrinth (in the public domain) for your use as a caregiver and for your elder to enjoy. Choose a time and place where you can focus and "walk" your finger labyrinth without being disturbed.

For additional information on labyrinths or for purchasing labyrinths visit:

- http://www.veriditas.org: Inspiring transformation through the labyrinth experience. Also offers pilgrimages, workshops, and trainings about the labyrinth.
- https://www.ispiritual.com: "Walking the path of the heart"
- http://www.amazon.com/Chartres-Double-Finger-Labyrinth-Wood/dp/ B009KAY6UG

There's an App for That!

Finger Labyrinth HD can be found in app stores and offers many labyrinth designs to use.

The previous information is adapted with permission from material found on the http://www.veriditas.org website. It is used with permission from Veriditas.

USING FINGER LABYRINTHS FOR MEDITATION

By Sr. Mary Jo Chaves
Spiritual Director and Retreat Leader
Franciscan Spiritual Center, Milwaukie, Oregon
http://www.francisspctr.com

Place your labyrinth in front of you or comfortably on your lap. Enter the entrance of your finger labyrinth with the index finger of your non-dominant hand to begin your meditation through the finger labyrinth. If using your non-dominant hand is awkward or uncomfortable, you can use the index finger of your dominant hand or a stylus instead.

1. **Prepare**—Before you enter the labyrinth, reflect on your life right now. What is it that seems to be welling up inside you at this present moment in your life? Let this pondering take root in your inner being.
2. **Enter**—Trace the pattern of the labyrinth with your finger or stylus. Simply follow the path and listen. Stop at times to rest if you choose. Let go of burdens, ideas, the need to control. Remember, all things on your walk will instruct. You won't get lost. Trust the path.
3. **Center**—When you reach the center, linger and stay as long as you like. This is a place to listen to the still small voice of the Divine and receive.

Words may not be given to you. At some level, conscious or subconscious, your being is receiving the message.
4. **Return**—When you are ready, begin your journey back. Be aware of your feelings, your energy, and insights or images. Let your being express gratitude for your walk.

This meditation is ongoing and may find its way into your life outside the actual time you spend with your finger labyrinth. The important thing to remember is that meditating with the labyrinth is a parable for life. At times you may feel confident of the path, and, at other times, you simply may be invited to trust the path by tracing it slowly and with intention, one small movement at a time. In the end, you will arrive at the center, encountering the Divine who is already there waiting for you. Let the meditation be analogous to going on a pilgrimage. Above all, be gentle with yourself. Enjoy the journey!

Copyright © 2016 by Sr. Mary Jo Chaves. Reprinted with permission.

SPIRITUAL REFLECTIONS ON LOVING THE REAL WHEN MOM DOESN'T KNOW WHO I AM

By Mary Jo Saavedra

It was a sunny Saturday morning in the spring of 2011. Lilacs were in full bloom, casting their heady sweet smell through my mom's bedroom window at the residential memory care home where she resided. This day, as I walked into Mom's room, her face lit up with real joy in seeing me. I, in return, felt the familiar love for this amazing woman wash over me. I hugged her tightly and asked how she had slept the night before. Then I commented how heavenly the lilacs smelled! She replied enthusiastically, "Yes, they smell lovely! They are my favorite flower—and what do you do here?" My breath caught and I actually could feel my heart crack.

I knew lilacs were Mom's favorite flower; she had covered every available surface in our home with fresh lilac clippings in the early days of every spring when I was growing up. In fact, I knew most everything about her, and she had known everything about me—until this day.

The lapse of recognizing me lasted only a few moments on that particular day but defined for me how the process of being with her required me to lean into meeting her where she was in her dementia experience. In an interview cited on Caring.com, geriatrician Dr. Bill Thomas explains this profound insight that can help us to shift our sense of loss and pain into a meaningful spiritual practice. The practice can ultimately sustain us in joy while we continue the fragile relationship with a parent in advanced memory loss. He says:

> So someone says, *"I go to see my mom, she doesn't know my name. I hold her hand, she doesn't hold my hand back. I talk to her, she doesn't speak to me."* There are a lot of people dealing with that, and here's a way to make sense out of it: Your mom is giving you a chance to take it to the next level, to give love simply and purely on the basis of love and compassion, not on the basis of asking, *"What am I getting back out of this?"* It's an advanced spiritual practice.
>
> Part of the reason why "elderhood," or old age exists is to help lead us toward this advanced kind of spiritual understanding. I have compassion for people who are facing a mother or father who doesn't recognize them any-more—that's pretty tough—and, of course, I've seen it as a geriatrician for years. But there's still more to learn, and your parent can still teach you. It's just different. And that takes some getting used to.[18]

So, what does "different" look like? How do we do this spiritual prac-tice? Will we ever get used to being "different" with our own parent? There are as many answers to these questions as there are people. "Different" will be unique for each of us. But the one thing that will be constant, that will define the action as a spiritual practice, is our willingness to say "Yes" to showing up—to choosing, time after time, to spiritually show up and meet our elder where he is in his experience. By doing this, we free ourselves from suffering and enter into what Buddha calls "Beginner's Mind," or what St. Thérèse of Lisieux calls the "Little Way." This mindset or "way" is a practice in which we set what we know aside, surrender, and enter into the experience as new, as a place of growth and learning, a place of deep connection and awareness, a place we come with love and imperfection.

My mother continued to hold my spiritual hand and teach me this concept. She showed me how to live with the real, where she was in the moment, and, ultimately, to be with her as she transitioned into death. The journey was not easy, and I admit that pleading prayers for her release from this world were my constant companions as I observed her in terrors of hallucinations, time travel, frustration, and fear—brutal symptoms of her Lewy Body dementia. Second only to Alzheimer's disease as the most common dementia, Lewy Body tears through the brain. But daily, almost hourly, precious moments would unfold to keep me present to her needs as well as present to my own needs.

Part of being present to "what is" comes in the spiritual practice of being—be-ing together, being present, and being aware—finding a point of inspiration with your elder that allows you to simply be present to him where he is. If "being" takes on a presence of activity or curiosity on your part, don't be surprised if an elder's childhood interests emerge to live again, or things you never knew about her are shared in stories, or perhaps new fantasies unfold in his imagination that are not tethered to anything concrete in his past experience other than a long-forgotten dream or childhood fear. In fact, finding new ways to be together can take on interesting and even exciting dimensions. Remember, simply through your presence you have already chosen "Yes." And this is gift enough.

THE NIGHT IS A PERSON

By Bill Gottlieb, CHC
Best-selling health author
http://billgottliebhealth.com

You could think, walking at dusk in the woods,
the light leaking out of the day,
your mind suffused with sudden angers,
as if every branch you see is whipping across your eyes,
as if all the trees are people who had tried to dominate you,
taller, older—that the night is like a person.
He puts the new moon in a slot and wins the stars
and then loses them,
and you have to pay for his passage
through all those hours of air.
He calls you from far away and complains he can't hear you.
He likes to make you stumble, he likes
you looking over your shoulder, wondering what's next.
But the night isn't a person, or at least not that person,
not your father, who has told you once again—
his broken hip mending, his collapsed lung hanging in there,
that damned daughter never calling,
twenty dollars in his bank account until the next Treasury check,
teeth gone, seeing double, tremor worse—
that he couldn't have done it without you,
stopped lying, lived on, lived on as the old man
you love helplessly, like a seed loves ground,
his body, just an hour or so ago, thousands of miles east,
steeped in the black conclusion
that hasn't yet arrived where you live
but definitely will.

WHEN YOU SIT WITH ME

By Regina G. Roman

When you sit with me
I am an icon,
mirror into the soul,
reflecting your phenomenal human nature.

Tell me what you see.

Your smiles and tears
etched momentarily into my heart
create an outline of soul.

Your memories
invoking ancient pigments of thought
are placed briefly on the white board of my mind.

Your words
puddle and push both intense opaque color
and forgiving transparent washes into emerging layers,
until awareness
is drawn to the perfect whole.

Your story,
the somber shadows
nestled against the halo's golden glow,
is every saint's image.

When you sit with me
I am an icon,
window to heaven,
allowing the luminous divine nature in you
to be seen.

This is how I listen.

WEEP NOT FOR ME

By Kym Croft Miller

Weep not for me
For I am not gone
To be with me
You have only to look
With new eyes
And to listen
With fresh ears

I am in the smile
Of an eager baby
As I am in the shuffle
Of an old man

Hear my whisper in the whir
Of sun-drunk bees,
My chuckle in the pulse
Of a tumbling stream

And when you least expect it
Find me there

There in the crumbling stones of a castle
There in an Irish song, sung deep and slow
There among shadows and light
There in the space between all sound
There I am

Weep not for me
For I am not gone
I am with you now, only everywhere

Glossary

Activities of Daily Living (ADLs): There are six basic ADLs: functional mobility, bathing and showering, dressing, self-feeding, personal hygiene, and toilet hygiene. An individual's ability to perform ADLs is important for determining what type of LTC and assistance the individual needs.

Acute Rehab Hospital (or Inpatient Rehabilitation Facility): Similar to nursing homes, these facilities provide doctor-ordered medical care for people who have suffered an injury or illness but no longer need to be in the hospital and are not yet able to return home because they need intensive rehabilitative therapy. Acute rehab hospitals typically provide the therapy several hours a day, so the patient must be medically stable enough to handle that level of rehabilitation. Such an intensive level of therapy usually is not available at many skilled nursing facilities or nursing homes.

Adult Daycare Facility: Adult daycare facilities provide drop-in activities for elders in a safe environment. Typically open during daytime hours on Monday through Friday, these facilities often feature crafts, music, dining, and other forms of entertainment in their offerings. Some offer day trips, health and medical services, and support for elders with Alzheimer's and dementia. Some even provide transportation. If an elder is being treated medically while at these facilities, part or most of the cost may be covered by Medicaid or LTC insurances. This is not always the case, however, so it pays to check into this carefully.

Adult Foster Care Home: Adult care or adult foster care homes are single-family residences offering a "home-like" environment for between two and ten elders; the maximum number is determined by each state. Typically, the owners of the home or the hired care providers live in the home with the residents. Adult foster care homes are considerably less expensive than assisted living facilities, but, of course, they have fewer amenities. Nonetheless, elders who dislike large facilities often enjoy the smaller, home-like environment of adult care homes. The services vary from one home to another, and there isn't a "standard." Choosing the right adult foster care home requires doing your homework and going in with a checklist of the services and type of care you want to experience. Most provide supervised custodial care, meals, and laundry services. Most expect the elder to be ambulatory and to be able to perform personal hygiene with minimal supervision. Some allow wheelchairs, whereas others don't. Some adult care homes are licensed to dispense medications, and others may provide more extensive medical support (although this level of support is less common in adult care homes). They may provide transportation to medical appointments and outside activities, although not all do.

Advance Healthcare Directive (or Advance Directive): Gives instructions for future life-sustaining treatment and typically includes a HCPOA, which names the "healthcare agent" who will make healthcare decisions for an individual in the event the individual is unable to communicate.

Each state typically will have its own statutory document that should be used. If your state uses a statutory document (meaning a document that is always in a particular form under state law), you often can get this from your doctor. Also, most estate planning and elder law attorneys include this form for their clients as part of their overall planning process.

All adults, regardless of their current health status, are recommended to complete this document. **Keep it with the rest of your estate planning documents (your trust, will, and DPOA), and giving a copy to your primary care provider is a good idea.** This document will *not* guide emergency medical personnel, but the document does guide inpatient treatment decisions if it is available.

An advance healthcare directive is sometimes confused with a living will. They are similar documents in that both give instructions regarding life-sustaining treatment, but the advance healthcare directive also typically includes the HCPOA in the document. If your state uses a living will, you probably also will need to complete a separate HCPOA. You should consult with your estate planning attorney regarding what documents are required and appropriate in your state. You can download your state's advance directive by visiting http://www.caringinfo.org.

Aging at Home or Aging in Place: This definition is easy, because it's just as it sounds: You are living independently in your home. You may have relatives or friends living with you, but you are still living at home. Eventually, you also may bring in other people to support and enable you to stay in your home as long as possible.

Aging Life Care Manager (ALCM): ALCMs are aging experts who work with older adults and their adult children and loved ones to develop holistic aging plans and programs addressing all aspects of aging. They are advocates for elders and caregivers and they are "age" navigators whose primary goal is to define an approach to aging that supports maximum capable independence for the elder. Typically, ALCMs have a health, social services, or gerontology background, and most hold advanced degrees. Certified ALCMs have met rigorous professional standards, passed the ALCM® exam, and agreed to adhere to strict principles when giving care-planning advice. See http://www.aginglifecare.org.

Assisted Living Facility (or Assisted Living Home): Assisted living "homes" or facilities can range from independent living to "full-care" living. Some facilities focus on a specific level or type of support, whereas others provide continuous care—from independent living to medical care and memory care units. Typically, twenty or more (could be several hundred) elders reside at any one time in an assisted living facility. Elders may move to assisted living for several reasons: They no longer want to maintain a home or apartment; they enjoy engaging with a larger group of elders; they enjoy planned group activities and trips; they want some or all meals prepared; they want or need an increasing level of custodial and/or medical care; they need transportation; they feel safer; or it's become too expensive or impractical to have full-time help at home.

Beneficiary: A person named to receive property after the death of the property owner. A beneficiary is typically named in a last will and testament, a trust, in a beneficiary designation on a retirement account or insurance policy, or in a "Transfer on Death" or "Payable on Death" designation on certain types of financial accounts. *Note*: A beneficiary designation overrides a will.

Brokerage House/Firm: A financial institution that facilitates the buying and selling of financial securities such as stocks, bonds, and mutual funds. Brokerage companies generally are paid by commission on the products you invest in and by transaction fees.

Case Managers: These individuals work for insurance companies. Their main role is to interpret and apply the benefits of that insurance to its members. They often have large caseloads of members to advocate for and support.

Certified Financial Planner (CFP®): CFP®s have met rigorous professional standards, passed the CFP® exam, and agreed to adhere to strict principles when giving financial advice. They may or may not manage money.

Certified Public Accountant (CPA): A person who has passed the Uniform Certified Public Accountant Exam and has met additional state education and experience requirements in accounting and tax preparation.

Certified Senior Advisor (CSA): Professionals addressing many different needs of elders including care managers, accountants, real estate people, attorneys, financial advisors, and others who have chosen to focus their attention on aging adults. They become certified through the Society of Certified Senior Advisors by attending classes, passing an extensive exam, and maintaining their certification through required continuing education. See http://www.csa.us.

Conservator: A person appointed by a court to take care of the finances of a "protected person," who is someone the court has determined needs assistance with the management of finances and assets. Most conservators are family members, or sometimes friends, who agree to serve. There are also professionals who will serve in this capacity, or they can be appointed by the court, if there is no family member or friend willing or able to serve.

Conservatorship: A matter in which a court-appointed individual, the "conservator," takes care of the financial and legal matters of someone the court deems needs assistance with such management. A conservatorship is typically required when someone becomes incapacitated and does not have proper planning in place (a DPOA or a trust), which would allow her assets to be managed on her behalf without court intervention. The court is required to be involved at that point in order for someone to have legal authority to manage the incapacitated person's assets.

Continuing Care Retirement Community (CCRC): The traditional model of a CCRC is a facility that offers four levels of care: independent living; non-medical support or "assisted living"; medical care; and memory care. CCRCs often but not always require a buy-in that can be anywhere from $100,000 to $1 million, together with a monthly fee of anywhere from $3,000 to $7,000. The buy-in fee *may be* partially refundable, depending upon whether the fees have been applied to advanced levels of care.

Corneal Implant: A damaged or diseased cornea can be replaced with donated corneal tissue, either entirely or partially, through a surgical procedure.

Custodial Care: If you are aging at home and you find you are struggling to accomplish daily tasks such as dressing, bathing, cooking, shopping, cleaning, and getting to appointments, you might hire an agency or individual to provide "custodial" care or personal care. Custodial care providers do not provide medical care. Keep in mind that, if you hire an individual rather than hiring someone through an agency, you may become, from a tax perspective, an "employer" and, therefore, responsible for payroll taxes and insurance.

Decedent: A person who has died.

Defibrillator (ICD): An implantable cardioverter defibrillator (ICD) is a small device placed in the chest or abdomen. Doctors use the device to help treat irregular heartbeats called arrhythmias. An ICD uses electrical pulses or shocks to help control life-threatening arrhythmias, especially those that can cause sudden cardiac arrest.

Dental Implant (also known as an endosseous implant or fixture): This is a surgical component that interfaces with the bone of the jaw or skull to support a dental prosthesis such as a crown, bridge, denture, or facial prosthesis or to act as an orthodontic anchor.

Discharge Planners: Professionals whose role is to facilitate an effective and appropriate discharge from the hospital to home and/or another setting. They work with insurance case managers and other health care providers in the hospital to ensure a smooth transition from hospital to home, nursing home, and/or another community setting.

Doctor of Osteopathy (DO): A DO is a fully trained and licensed doctor who has attended and graduated from a U.S. osteopathic medical school. The major difference between osteopathic (DO) and allopathic (MD) doctors is that some osteopathic doctors provide manual medicine therapies such as cranial-sacral work, spinal manipulation, or massage therapy, as part of their treatment, whereas MDs do not.

Durable Power of Attorney (DPOA): A document in which someone, "the principal," names an "agent" or "attorney-in-fact" to manage her assets and finances. This can be created to be effective immediately or to have effect upon incapacity (a "springing" POA). A DPOA no longer has any legal effect after the death of the principal. A DPOA can be drafted by your estate planning or elder law attorney to address your specific situation.

Estate: All property and debts belonging to a person. Everyone has an "estate," even if it is very small.

Executor, Personal Representative, or Administrator: A person named in a last will and testament (personal representative or executor) or appointed by a court (administrator) to oversee the administration of the estate of someone who has passed away. An administrator is appointed by the court when the decedent did not have a last will and testament. There are many considerations that go into choosing the appropriate person to serve as personal representative. Your estate planning attorney should guide you through this choice when you are designing your estate plan.

Family Practitioner: Physician trained to provide care to an individual and all family members regardless of age, gender, or medical diagnosis.

Fee-only Advisor: An investment advisor who charges you based on a percentage of your assets under management (AUM). He does not receive any commissions on products you use or receive any other fees for your investments.

Fiduciary: A person who has a legal duty to act solely in another party's interest. A personal representative, executor, administrator, trustee, conservator, guardian, healthcare agent, and attorney-in-fact are all types of fiduciaries.

Finance/Billing Advocates: These individuals work in the area of finance and billing. They can coordinate with insurance case managers to facilitate the accurate accounting of healthcare charges and assist with interpreting an elder's healthcare bills. They also can advocate on an elder's behalf regarding billing within health systems.

Financial Power of Attorney: See "Durable Power of Attorney."

Geriatric Psychiatrist (also known as geropsychiatrist or geripsychiatrist): Doctor of medicine (MD) specializing in the area of psychiatry who deals with the study, prevention, and treatment of mental disorders in the elderly.

Geriatrician: Internist or family physician specially trained in the care of older adults (generally defined as seventy-five years of age and older). This type of MD tends to focus on complex medical and social issues related to aging.

Gerontology: The multidisciplinary study of aging that encompasses the medical, biological, social, religious/spiritual, financial, and legal effects on people as they age. Those with academic degrees in this discipline are called **gerontologists**. Not MDs, these professionals may be involved in research within the industry, consult with businesses as population segment specialists, teach at universities, or provide direct support to elders through private and public agencies for managing various aspects of aging. Some gerontologists are also certified aging life care managers, certified senior advisors, and more.

Geropsychologist: A doctor of psychology (PhD) devoted to the study of aging and the provision of clinical services related to mental and behavioral health for older adults.

Guardianship: A matter in which a court-appointed and supervised individual, the "guardian," makes day-to-day decisions for a "protected person," someone the court has determined needs assistance with those decisions due to the potential for harm to herself or others, most often due to incapacity or some other cognitive impairment. The appointed guardian is responsible for decisions such as living situations, management of health care, or advance funeral arrangements. A guardianship is typically required when someone becomes incapacitated and does not have proper planning in place (HCPOA, HIPAA authorization, advance healthcare directive), which would allow another person to manage the care of the incapacitated person without court intervention.

Healthcare Power of Attorney (HCPOA): A document in which an "agent" is named to make healthcare decisions for an individual, the "principal." If you are in a state that uses an advance healthcare directive, the HCPOA is typically included in that document. Otherwise, your estate planning attorney should include this document in your estate plan.

Healthcare Representative or Healthcare Agent: This is a person named in an advance directive or a HCPOA to manage the healthcare decisions of the principal in the event she is unable to communicate or is otherwise incapacitated.

Health Insurance Portability and Accountability Act (HIPAA): This act was passed by Congress in 1996; it limits access to private healthcare information. A properly drafted estate plan should include a HIPAA authorization and release, so the principal's loved ones can have access to necessary medical information.

Heir: A person legally entitled to inherit assets of a decedent, based on state statute and when there is no other planning in place, such as a will or trust. For example, a child is typically an heir of her widowed father. If the father has no estate plan (i.e., no will or trust), the child will inherit based on the laws of intestacy in the state where the father lived. The father can, however, disinherit the child or include additional beneficiaries if he creates a last will and testament or a trust in which he specifies how he wants his assets to be distributed.

Home Health Care: As you age, you may find that aging at home is best for you; however, at some point, you may require in-home support for medical issues. For example, you may need to have someone provide injections, oversee medication management, offer wound treatment, and/or monitor an acute or ongoing illness. This level of support is provided by home healthcare providers.

Hospice or End-of-Life Care: Hospice or end-of-life care is provided to qualified Medicare recipients whose life expectancy is six months or less. Through the hospice program, a team of healthcare professionals and volunteers provide medical, psychological, and spiritual support at home, in hospitals, in assisted care, at hospice centers, and skilled nursing facilities. The goal of hospice comfort care is to provide peace and dignity to those who are dying and to their loved ones.

Hospice and Palliative Medicine Specialist: Prevents and relieves suffering of patients who have a serious illness or who have only a short time to live.

Hospitalist: Physician specializing in hospital care who can coordinate and provide treatment in place of a PCP when the patient is hospitalized.

Incapacity: A lack or the loss of the ability to take care of oneself.

Inpatient Rehabilitation Facility (IRF): Similar to nursing homes, these facilities provide doctor-ordered medical care for people who have suffered an injury or illness, no longer need to be in the hospital, but are unable to return home because they need intensive rehabilitative therapy. IRFs typically provide therapy several hours a day, and the patient must be medically stable enough to handle that level of rehabilitation. Such an intensive level of therapy usually is not available at many SNFs or nursing homes; SNFs can be an interim step for patients who need skilled nursing care but are not yet ready for acute rehabilitation. In essence, patients can use the SNF step to gain strength before moving to the IRF. The discharge planner at the local hospital is the best resource for IRFs in the community.

Internist: Physician who most often cares for adults and their medical needs. Patients usually range from older adolescents through older adults. Some internists continue to study an area of sub-specialty (neurology, orthopedics, pulmonology, etc.).

Intestacy: Intestacy means, simply, dying without having a will in place. The practical result of intestacy is that state statute will determine where and to whom the assets will pass. This may or may not match the wishes of the decedent. For example, James Dean's estate passed to the long-estranged father who abandoned him, because he had no will or trust in place.

Investment Advisor: A fee-only or commission-based money manager. This person will advise on investing in stocks, bonds, and other securities. Should be registered with the Securities and Exchange Commission (SEC) or your state's Division of Finance and Corporate Securities.

Investment Advisor Representative (IAR): An advisor whose main responsibility is to provide investment advice. IARs can only provide advice on topics on which they have passed the appropriate exams. An IAR must be registered with the proper state authorities. Many hold a Certified Financial Planner (CFP®) or Chartered Financial Analyst (CFA®) designation.

Last Will and Testament: A legal document that names beneficiaries of property of a decedent and a person responsible for overseeing the distribution of the property. The responsible person is called an "executor" or "personal representative." Wills only have legal effect at death.

Legacy Letter: Also known as a "wisdom will" or an "ethical will." It is a document written with the intention of sharing values, life lessons, hopes and dreams, and a heartfelt expression of what truly matters most in life with family and/or friends. This is not a legal document.

Living Will: *See* Advance Healthcare Directive.

Long-term Care (LTC): This is a "catch-all" term for programs and facilities that support assisted-living including assisted care homes, adult foster care, nursing homes, acute care facilities, rehab facilities, etc.

Minimum Required Distribution (MRD): You cannot keep retirement funds in your account indefinitely. The Internal Revenue Service (IRS) requires a minimum distribution from your account when you reach the age of seventy and a half. The required minimum distribution is a calculated number. The IRS website at https://www.irs.gov/Retirement-Plans has tools and calculators for determining the correct amount. Roth IRAs do not require withdrawals until after the death of the owner.

Naturopathic Doctor (ND): NDs practice what is called naturopathy, a distinct system of primary health care that emphasizes prevention and the self-healing process through the use of natural therapies.

Nurse Practitioner (NP): An NP is qualified to treat certain medical conditions without the direct supervision of a doctor. NPs diagnose and treat health conditions with an emphasis on disease prevention and health management.

Occupational Therapist (OT): Highly trained professional who works with people to enhance their ability to engage in everyday activities. The OT does this by teaching new techniques to do everyday activities, providing equipment that facilitates independence, and recommending environmental (or home) modifications that support independence. OTs work in a variety of settings such as hospitals, nursing homes, private practices, outpatient clinics, and home health agencies.

Ombudsman: Professional who advocates for residents of LTC facilities. Each state's ombudsman can typically be found by searching online for "ombudsman [state]." States also require that the ombudsman's name and contact information be posted in plain sight in adult care facilities.

Pacemaker: This small device, when surgically placed in the chest or abdomen, helps to control arrhythmias (abnormal heart rhythms.) This device uses electrical pulses to prompt the heart to beat at a normal rate.

Paid on Death (POD) Account: A type of account that will distribute all money to the designated pay-on-death beneficiary. This type of account can avoid probate and gives the beneficiary immediate access to the money.

Palliative Care: The goal of palliative care is to relieve patients of the pain and stress of serious illness, with a goal to improve quality of life for the patient and his or her family. Palliative care is delivered holistically through a team of doctors and nurses, social workers, pharmacists, chaplains, and others. Whereas palliative care is always incorporated into hospice care and often thought of as end-of-life care or care for someone who cannot be cured, it also can be provided to patients with a non-life-threatening but serious illness, as it can be very helpful in eliminating pain and emotional distress.

Personal Representative (PR): See Executor.

Phishing Scam: The attempt to acquire sensitive information such as usernames, passwords, and credit card details (and sometimes, indirectly, money) by masquerading as a trustworthy entity in an electronic communication.

Physical Therapist (PT): Highly educated, state-licensed healthcare professional who can help patients reduce pain and improve or restore mobility through exercises, manipulation, massage, and other modalities—in many cases without expensive surgery and often reducing the need for long-term use of prescription medications and their side effects. In addition, the PT works with individuals to prevent the loss of mobility before it occurs by developing fitness- and wellness-oriented programs for healthier and more active lifestyles. PTs work in a variety of settings.

Physician Orders for Life-Sustaining Treatment (POLST): This is a companion to an advance healthcare directive or a living will, intended for persons of any age who have a serious illness. The POLST gives medical orders for current treatment and will guide inpatient treatment. Unlike the advance directive or a living will, the POLST *will* guide emergency medical personnel, if it is available.

Currently, POLST forms are available in more than half of the states in the United States, and they use various names—MOLST, POST, and COLST. To learn about the POLST form in your state or to find out if your state is developing one, check out http://www.polst.org/programs-in-your-state. In states where they are available, POLST forms can be obtained from primary care physicians, who must sign and register the form in the POLST national database. POLST forms are typically required to be printed on a specific color of paper. Also, post the complete POLST form in a public location such as the refrigerator, so it is easily accessible in the event of an emergency.

Physician's Assistant (PA): A highly trained, educated, and qualified medical professional who assists physicians and carries out routine clinical procedures under the supervision of physicians.

Power of Attorney (POA): A legal document giving someone the authority to sign documents and conduct transactions on another person's behalf. POAs are common estate planning documents; many people sign a financial power of attorney, also known as a durable power of attorney (DPOA), to give a friend or family member the power to conduct financial transactions for them if they become incapacitated. People also commonly sign healthcare powers of attorney (HCPOA) to give someone else the authority to make medical decisions if they are unable to do so. You also might give someone POA to act in a particular transaction if you cannot do it yourself, such as signing documents at a real estate closing when you are out of town.

Probate: The process of settling a decedent's estate under the supervision of a court. Probate is necessary if someone dies without an estate plan in place, or if she passes away with a will-only plan (i.e., no trust in place).

Resource Coordinators: Individuals hired by a healthcare system to advocate for and help patients navigate their system. They also can suggest and connect people with community resources for support and education.

Respite Care: Respite care offers caregivers (volunteers or relatives) the opportunity to take a break from their caregiving duties. Some assisted care facilities have extra rooms so an elder can stay just for a few days. Many home healthcare agencies also provide help. Adult daycare centers can relieve care providers during the day. Call your faith community and/or senior center to find out if there are volunteers who will help with respite care. If you are under hospice care, Medicare and/or Medicaid may cover respite care. For more on respite care, check out http://www.helpguide.org/articles/caregiving/respite-care.htm.

Reverse Mortgage: A home loan that provides cash payments based on home equity. Normally, the loan does not need to be repaid until the death of the homeowner, or until the homeowner sells or moves out of the home.

Shared Housing: An extension to "aging at home" is aging in a home that an elder buys or rents with other elders. Typically, the relationship is defined through a legal contract. Think of *The Golden Girls* sitcom. This type of living environment is often for independent elders who simply want to decrease their cost of living and/or to create a life that is more socially engaged. However, some elders who are more dependent upon custodial or healthcare support may also come together as a group to live together and share needed support.

Skilled Nursing Facility (SNF) and Nursing Home: The terms *skilled nursing facility* and *nursing home* are often used interchangeably, but they are not the same. If your elder qualifies for intensive care following a stay at a hospital, Medicare will only pay for a SNF facility. The guidelines for qualifying as a SNF require a higher number of skilled nurses and doctors than a nursing home. However, many, if not most, nursing homes do qualify as SNFs. You can acquire a list of certified facilities in your area from your medical insurance provider.

Stockbroker: An employee or agent who works for a brokerage house that charges a fee or commission for executing investment and trade orders for the investor.

Trust: A private legal document that controls the management of property and assets during each stage of life—while alive and well, during incapacity, and at death. A trust is a contract, and it takes effect immediately upon signing. Assets in a properly drafted, funded, and maintained trust will avoid having to go through the probate process, which often can save families time, money, and hassle.

Trustee: A trustee is the person in charge of protecting, managing, and distributing the assets held in a trust. A successor trustee is the person who will step in to serve if the initial trustee cannot or will not serve.

Vigiling: Quietly waiting, praying, and just being at the bedside of a sick or dying person. Volunteer vigilers are available in some areas if a person is alone during a major illness or during the end of life.

Village to Village Network (VtV): The VtV Network is a national peer-to-peer network that aids in improving management and coordination of a "village." Villages are groups of people who come together to coordinate access to services and to support one another in aging in place. http://vtvnetwork.org.

Virtual Retirement Community (VRC): VRCs are communities formed by seniors through contracts or agreements created to support aging at home through a community model. VRCs help create a close-knit community and access to services that may be needed when aging at home (e.g., transportation, home health care, home repair, etc.). The services may be provided by members of the VRC, by volunteers, and/or by paid providers who are recommended and screened by the community. The physical models of VRCs range from elders living in their home and forming the virtual community with others nearby but not necessarily in the exact same neighborhood to VRCs with entire neighborhoods specifically built for elders who want to create a VRC.

Notes

CHAPTER 3

1. Carol B. Bursack, "Do Parents Really Want to Live with Their Adult Children?" AgingCare.com, accessed October 24, 2015, http://www.agingcare.com/Articles/parents-living-with-adult-children-152285.htm.

CHAPTER 5

1. M. Jane Mohler, "Depression in Elders," *Elder Care: A Resource for Interprofessional Providers* (Tucson: University of Arizona Center on Aging, 2015), accessed October 29, 2015, https://nursingandhealth.asu.edu/sites/default/files/depression.pdf.
2. "What Is Depression?" National Institute of Mental Health, last modified October 29, 2015, https://www.nimh.nih.gov/health/topics/depression/index.shtml.
3. "How Much Sleep Do You Need?" National Sleep Foundation, last modified October 29, 2015, https://sleepfoundation.org/excessivesleepiness/how-sleep-works/how-much-sleep-do-we-really-need.
4. U.S. Institute of Medicine Committee on Sleep Medicine and Research, "Extent and Health Consequences of Chronic Sleep Loss and Sleep Disorders," in *Sleep Disorders and Sleep Deprivation: An Unmet Public Health Problem*, H. R. Colten and B. M. Altevogt, eds. (Washington, DC: National Academies Press, 2006), accessed October 29, 2015, http://www.ncbi.nlm.nih.gov/books/NBK19961/.
5. "The 90+ Study," last modified October 29, 2015, http://www.mind.uci.edu/research/90plus-study.
6. Center for Substance Abuse Treatment, "Substance Abuse among Older Adults: An Invisible Epidemic," chapter in *Treatment Improvement Protocol (TIP) Series* (Rockville, MD: U.S. Substance Abuse and Mental Health Services Administration, 1998), accessed October 30, 2015, http://www.ncbi.nlm.nih.gov/books/NBK64422.

7. Richard A. Friedman, "A Rising Tide of Substance Abuse," *New York Times*, April 29, 2013, accessed October 30, 2015, http://newoldage.blogs.nytimes.com/2013/04/29/a-rising-tide-of-mental-distress/?_r=0.

8. "The 90+ Study," last modified October 30, 2015, http://www.mind.uci.edu/research/90plus-study.

9. Carl W. Cotman, "Exercise Builds Brain Health," last modified October 30, 2015, http://www.mind.uci.edu/alzheimers-disease/articles-of-interest/behaviors-mindfulness-biomarkets-stem-cells-other-dementia/exercise-builds-brain-health/.

10. Joseph Campbell, *A Joseph Campbell Companion: Reflections on the Art of Living* (San Anselmo, CA: Joseph Campbell Foundation, 2011).

11. Johann Wolfgang von Goethe, *Torquato Tasso*, Act 1, sc. 11 (1790).

12. Atul Gawande, *Being Mortal: Medicine and What Matters in the End* (New York: Metropolitan Books, 2014), 44.

13. Gu Quiping, Charles F. Dillon, and Vicki L. Burt, "Prescription Drug Use Continues to Increase," *National Center for Health Statistics Data Brief* 42 (September 2010), accessed October 30, 2015, http://www.cdc.gov/nchs/data/databriefs/db42.htm.

14. "What Vaccines Are Recommended for You," Centers for Disease Control and Prevention, last modified October 29, 2015, http://www.cdc.gov/vaccines/adults/rec-vac/index.html?s_cid=cs_650.

15. Centers for Medicare and Medicaid Services, *Medicare and You: 2015* (Washington, D.C.: U.S. Department of Health and Human Services, 2015), 15.

16. With special thanks to Dr. Paul Glassman, DDS, MA, MBA, University of the Pacific Arthur A. Dugoni School of Dentistry, and Dr. Gregory J. Folse, DDS, Outreach Dentistry, Lafayette, LA.

17. A. A. El-Solh, C. Pietrantoni, A. Bhat, M. Okada, J. Zambon, A. Aquilina, and E. Berbary, "Colonization of Dental Plaques: A Reservoir of Respiratory Pathogens for Hospital-Acquired Pneumonia in Institutionalized Elders," *Chest* 126 (November 2004): 1575–82, accessed October 26, 2015, http://www.ncbi.nlm.nih.gov/pubmed/15539730.

18. P. J. Pussinen, G. Alfthan, H. Rissanen, et al., "Antibodies to Periodontal Pathogens and Stroke Risk," *Stroke* 35 (2004): 2020–23.

19. Department of Health and Human Services, *Oral Health in America: A Report of the Surgeon General* (Bethesda, MD: National Institute of Dental and Craniofacial Research, 2000), accessed October 26, 2015, http://profiles.nlm.nih.gov/ps/retrieve/ResourceMetadata/NNBBJT.

20. J. F. Moellar and N. A. Mathiowetz, *Prescribed Medicines: A Summary of Use and Expenditures for Medicare Beneficiaries* (Rockville, MD: U.S. Department of Health and Human Services), Publication PHC 89-3448, 198.

21. J. A. Ship, S. R. Pillemer, and B. J. Baum, "Xerostomia and the Geriatric Patient," *Journal of the American Geriatric Society* 50 (2002): 535–43.

22. Centers for Disease Control and Prevention, *The State of Aging and Health in America 2013* (Atlanta: Centers for Disease Control and Prevention, 2013), accessed October 29, 2015, http://www.cdc.gov/features/agingandhealth/state_of_aging_and_health_in_america_2013.pdf.

23. National Conference of State Legislatures and AARP Public Policy Institute, "Aging in Place: A State Survey of Livability Policies and Practices," *In Brief* 190 (December 2011), accessed October 29, 2015, http://assets.aarp.org/rgcenter/ppi/livcom/ib190.pdf.

CHAPTER 6

1. Dr. Payne has repeated this aphorism many times, but it was originally uttered by Gwen London, former director of the Institute on Care at the End of Life at Duke University. The exact quote is actually, "Dying is a spiritual event with medical implications." Dr. Payne expanded the idea of the original quotation. See: John Swinton and Richard Payne, eds., "Christian Practices and the Art of Dying Faithfully," *Living Well and Dying Faithfully: Christian Practices for End-of-Life Care* (Grand Rapids, MI: Eerdmans Publishing Company, 2009), xv.

2. "Mastering Materialism," *The Hindu*, July 15, 2001, accessed October 26, 2015, http://www.thehindu.com/2001/07/15/stories/13150611.htm.

3. Atul Gawande, *Being Mortal: Medicine and What Matters in the End* (New York: Metropolitan Books, 2014), 25–26.

4. Richard Groves and Henriette Klauser, *The American Book of Dying: Lessons in Healing Spiritual Pain* (Berkeley, CA: Celestial Arts, 2005), 1.

5. This insightful question was first introduced to me by the late Dr. Tom Leimert, who headed the Oncology and Hermatology Department at Kaiser Sunnyside Hospital in Portland, Oregon, for many years. For other insights shared in this section, I am particularly indebted to the work of Dr. Atul Gawande and Dr. Angelo Volandes, whose books (listed in the bibliography) have provided guidance to me as well as to my colleagues.

6. Special thanks to Douglas Smith, MA, MS, MDiv (dougcsmith.com) for suggesting these questions.

7. Fr. Richard John Neuhaus, "Born toward Dying," *First Things*, February, 2009, accessed October 26, 2015, http://www.firstthings.com/article/2000/02/born-toward-dying.

8. Cf. Henri Nouwen, *The Wounded Healer: Ministry in Contemporary Society* (Los Angeles: Image Books, 1979), 91.

9. Special thanks to Jennifer Faustin, RN, CHPN, from the Kaiser Westside Medical Center, Hillsboro, Oregon, for this insight.

10. Thomas Long and Thomas Lynch, *The Good Funeral: Death, Grief, and the Community of Care* (Louisville, KY: Westminster John Knox Press, 2013), 58.

11. With gratitude to Fr. Richard Rutherford, CSC, Emeritus Professor of Theology at the University of Portland, for his contributions to my thinking on these topics over the past twenty-plus years.

12. Thomas Lynch, *The Undertaking*, Documentary, produced by Miri Navasky and Karen O'Connor (Arlington, VA: PBS/Frontline, 2007). Here is a longer quote from the transcript, to put the shorter quote in context: "We're among the first couple generations for whom the presence of the dead at their own funerals has become optional.

We saw people start organizing sort of these commemorative events to which everyone was invited but the dead guy. And I see that as probably not good news for the culture at large. Up until a couple generations ago, humans dealt with death by dealing with their dead, so that the way we processed mortality was by processing from one place to the other. And both the dead and the living have some distance to go when someone we love dies."

13. Steven R. Covey, *The Seven Habits of Highly Effective People* (New York: Simon and Schuster, 1989), 95.

14. Katy Butler, "What Broke My Father's Heart: How a Pacemaker Wrecked Our Family's Life," KatyButler.com Blog, August 5, 2012, http://katybutler.com/site/a-pacemaker-wrecks-a-familys-life.

15. JFS Chaplain, "Celebrating One Year of Death Café Southbury," Deathcafe.com Blog, n.d., http://deathcafe.com/blog/109.

16. Oregon Public Health Division, "2013 Death with Dignity Act Report," http://public.health.oregon.gov/ProviderPartnerResources/EvaluationResearch/DeathwithDignityAct/Documents/year16.pdf.

17. Thanks to hospice volunteer and good friend John Rose for these words from a poem he wrote that graces a plaque welcoming visitors to Legacy Hopewell House, an inpatient hospice facility in Portland, Oregon.

18. To read the complete interview, go to https://www.caring.com/interviews/interview-with-bill-thomas-about-pulling-the-plug-on-nursing-homes.

Bibliography

Anderson, Megory. *Sacred Dying: Creating Rituals for Embracing the End of Life.* New York: Marlowe & Company, 2001.

———. *Attending the Dying: A Handbook of Practical Guidelines.* New York: Morehouse Publishing, 2005.

Bell, Karen W. *Living at the End of Life: A Hospice Nurse Addresses the Most Common Questions.* New York: Sterling Publishing, 2010.

Bolen, Jean Shinoda. *Close to the Bone: Life-Threatening Illness as a Soul Journey.* Newburyport, MA: Cornari Press, 2007.

Bregman, Lucy, ed. *Death and Dying in World Religions.* Dubuque, IA: Kendall Hunt Publishing, 2009.

———. *Religion, Death and Dying.* Westport, CT: Praeger, 2009.

Buchanan, Missy. *Living with Purpose in a Worn-Out Body.* Nashville, TN: Upper Room Books, 2008.

Buettner, Dan. *The Blue Zones: Lessons for Living Longer from the People Who've Lived the Longest.* Washington, D.C.: National Geographic, 2010.

Bulce Hurme, Sally. *ABA/AARP Checklist for Family Survivors: A Guide to Practical and Legal Matters When Someone You Love Dies.* Chicago: American Bar Association, 2014.

———. *ABA/AARP Checklist for My Family: A Guide to My History, My Finances, and My Final Wishes.* Chicago: American Bar Association, 2015.

Bush, Karen M., Louise S. Machinist, and Jean McQuillin. *My House Our House: Living Far Better for Far Less in a Cooperative Household.* Pittsburgh: St. Lynn's Press, 2013.

Butler, Katy. *Knocking on Heaven's Door: The Path to a Better Way of Death.* New York: Scribner, 2013.

Byock, Ira. *Dying Well: Peace and Possibilities at the End of Life.* New York: Riverhead Books, 1998.

———. *The Four Things That Matter Most: A Book about Living.* Washington, D.C.: Free Press, 2004.

283

————. *The Best Care Possible: A Physician's Quest to Transform Care through the End of Life.* New York: Avery Trade, 2013.

Callanan, Maggie, and Patricia Kelley. *Final Gifts: Understanding the Special Awareness, Needs, and Communications of the Dying.* New York: Bantam Books, 1992.

Callanan, Maggie. *Final Journeys: A Practical Guide for Bringing Care and Comfort at the End of Life.* New York: Bantam, 2009.

Clifford, Denis. *Estate Planning Basics: What You Need to Know about Wills, Trusts and Avoiding Probate.* 8th ed. Berkeley, CA: Nolo, 2015.

Dass, Ram. *Still Here: Embracing Aging, Changing and Dying.* New York: Riverhead Books, 2000.

Delehanty, Hugh, and Elinor Ginzler. *Caring for Your Parents: The Complete Guide.* New York: Sterling, 2008.

Gawande, Atul. *Being Mortal: Medicine and What Matters in the End.* New York: Metropolitan Books, 2014.

Groves, Richard, and Henriette Klauser. *The American Book of Dying: Lessons in Healing Spiritual Pain.* Berkeley, CA: Celestial Arts, 2005.

Halifax, Joan. *Being with Dying: Cultivating Compassion and Fearlessness in the Presence of Death.* Boulder, CO: Shambhala Publications, 2008.

Harrold, Joan, and Joan Lynne. *Handbook for Mortals: Guidance for People Facing Serious Illness.* New York: Oxford University Press, 1999.

Houle, Marcy Cottrell, and Elizabeth Eckstrom. *The Gift of Caring: Saving Our Parents from the Perils of Modern Healthcare.* Lanham, MD: Taylor Trade Publishing, 2015.

Kramer, Kenneth. *The Sacred Art of Dying: How World Religions Understand Death.* Mahwah, NJ: Paulist Press, 1988.

Kübler-Ross, Elisabeth, and Ira Byock. *On Death and Dying: What the Dying Have to Teach Doctors, Nurses, Clergy and Their Own Families.* Reprint ed. New York: Scribner, 2014.

Kustenmacher, Tiki, and Lothar Seiwert. *How to Simplify Your Life: Seven Practical Steps to Letting Go of Your Burdens and Living a Happier Life.* New York: McGraw-Hill, 2006.

Lamm, Maurice. *The Jewish Way in Death and Mourning.* Revised ed. Flushing, NY: Jonathan David Publishers, 2012.

Levine, Carol. *Planning for Long-Term Care for Dummies.* Hoboken, NJ: Wiley, 2014.

Levine, Stephen. *A Year to Live: How to Live This Year as If It Were Your Last.* New York: Harmony Books, 1997.

Long, Thomas, and Thomas Lynch. *The Good Funeral: Death, Grief, and the Community of Care.* Louisville, KY: Westminster John Knox Press, 2013.

Loverde, Joy. *The Complete Eldercare Planner: Where to Start, Which Questions to Ask, and How to Find Help.* New York: Harmony, 2009.

Manteau-Rao, Marguerite. *Caring for a Loved One with Dementia.* Oakland, CA: New Harbinger Press, 2016.

Matthews, Joseph L. *Long-Term Care: How to Plan and Pay for It.* 10th ed. Berkeley, CA: Nolo, 2014.

McCullough, Dennis. *My Mother, Your Mother: Embracing "Slow Medicine," the Compassionate Approach to Caring for Your Aging Loved Ones.* New York: Harper Perennial, 2009.

Morris, Virginia. *How to Care for Aging Parents: A One-Stop Resource for All Your Medical, Financial, Housing, and Emotional Issues.* 3rd ed. Workman Publishing, 2014.

O'Rourke, Michelle. *Befriending Death: Henri Nouwen and a Spirituality of Dying.* Maryknoll, NY: Orbis Books, 2009.

Parkes, C. M., P. Laungani, and W. Young, eds. *Death and Bereavement across Cultures.* New York: Routledge, 1997.

Rinpoche, Sogyal. *The Tibetan Book of Living and Dying: Revised and Updated Edition.* New York: HarperOne, 2002.

Rohr, Richard. *Falling Upward: A Spirituality for the Two Halves of Life.* San Francisco: Jossey-Bass, 2011.

Siala, Mohamed Ebrahim. *Authentic Step-by-Step Illustrated Janazah Guide.* http://www.missionislam.com/knowledge/janazahstepbystep.htm.

Singh, Kathleen Dowling. *The Grace in Aging: Awaken as You Grow Older.* Somerville, MA: Wisdom Publications, 2014.

Swinton, John, and Richard Payne. *Living Well and Dying Faithfully: Christian Practices for End-of-Life Care.* Grand Rapids, MI: Eerdmans, 2009.

Thibault, Jane Marie, and Richard L. Morgan. *Pilgrimage into the Last Third of Life: Seven Gateways to Spiritual Growth.* Nashville, TN: Upper Room Books, 2012.

Vogt, Susan V. *Blessed by Less: Clearing Your Life of Clutter by Living Lightly.* Chicago: Loyola Press, 2013.

Volandes, Angelo. *The Conversation: A Revolutionary Plan for End-of-Life Care.* New York: Bloomsbury USA, 2015.

Ware, Bronnie. *The Top Five Regrets of the Dying: A Life Transformed by the Dearly Departing.* Carlsbad, CA: Hay House, 2012.

York, Sarah. *Remembering Well: Rituals for Celebrating Life and Mourning Death.* San Francisco: Jossey-Bass, 2000.

Index

401(k). *See* retirement accounts

403(b). *See* retirement accounts

90+ Study, University of California at Irvine, 158–59, 160

abuse, elder, 12, 85, 94, 144, 146–47

activities of daily living, 64, 65, 83, 106, 182, 192, 194, 195, 200

acute rehab hospitals. *See* inpatient rehabilitation facilities

addiction. *See* substance abuse

ADLs. *See* activities of daily living

adult day care, 66, 125, 128

adult foster care homes, 52, 79, 104, 105, 107–10, 113, 114, 193, 195, 208

adult protective services, 144, 146–47

advance directive, 14, 16, 17, 18, 19, 24, 176, 192, 229–31, 247

advance healthcare directive. *See* advance directive

after–life considerations, 215–17, 237–44

age–restricted communities, 81–82

aging life care manager, 199–201

aging–at–home specialists. *See* aging–in–place specialists

aging–in–place specialists, 75, 88, 98, 102

Al–Fatiha, 246

ALCM. *See* aging life care manager

ALF. *See* assisted living facility

Altman, Donald, 255–56

Alzheimer's disease, 203, 204–5

Anglican, 244

Area Agency on Aging, 35, 54, 108, 109, 133, 134

art therapy, 124, 127

assisted living facility, 52, 58, 64, 65, 104–7, 111–16, 193, 202

assisted living home. *See* assisted living facility

audiologist, 170–71

auto insurance, 63

Bahai, 245

beneficiaries, 17, 20, 23, 39, 42–43, 45, 63, 64

benefit period, 66, 197

benefits, 12, 19, 23–24, 31, 38–41, 45, 60–66, 72, 89, 103, 181–83, 211, 212, 214

blue zones, 120

bonds, 46, 47

brain disease, 201–07

breathwork specialist, 170

brokerage houses/firms, 46

Buddhist, 244

Buettner, Dan. *See* blue zones

burial, 216, 235, 237, 238, 239, 244

car, finding the. *See* transportation issues
case managers, 157, 199
Catholic, 244, 245
CCRC. *See* continuing care retirement center
celebration of life, 236, 239–41
Center for Contemplative Mind In Society, 254–55
certified financial planner, 68
certified public accountant, 43, 46, 48, 54, 64, 66, 67–68, 72
certified senior advisor, 270
CFP. *See* certified financial planner
Chaves, Sr. Mary Jo, 258, 260–61
checking and savings accounts, 45
checkups, 155, 179, 185, 189
chewing (mastication) problems, 186
cochlear implants, 191
collectibles, 36
companions, 89, 90, 123, 162, 173, 251–52
computers, elder friendly, 36
conservator, 12, 15, 16, 19, 53
contemplative practices, 254–55
continuing care retirement center, 104–7, 111–13, 116, 193, 202
corneal implants, 191
cost of care, 58, 91, 104
CPA. *See* certified public accountant
credit and debit card accounts, 51–52
credit counseling, 56–57, 72
credit reports, 50, 55–56, 72
cremation, 216–17, 235, 238–39
Creutzfeldt–Jakob dementia, 203
CSA. See certified senior advisor
custodial care provider, 89, 91, 93–95

daily money manager, 33, 54–55, 72
death café, 248–51
death with dignity, 249–51
debt, 19, 26, 56–58
dementia, 65, 101, 106, 116, 124, 128, 144, 164, 201–7, 248, 261–62
dental implants, 184, 188

dental issues, 185–86
dentistry, geriatric, 184–90
dentures, 186, 187–88
depression in elders, 103, 126, 135, 157, 159, 168, 201, 213
dietician, 160, 170
disability insurance, 61, 65
DMM. *See* daily money manager
DO. *See* doctor of osteopathy
doctor of osteopathy, 165, 192
document storage, 37–38
donating stuff, 140–41, 227
DPOA. *See* durable power of attorney
driving, when to stop. *See* transportation issues
dry mouth, 186, 190
durable power of attorney, 9, 15, 17

eating, healthy, 102–03, 126, 135, 155, 159–60
Eden Alternative, 104, 126, 161
elder law attorney, 12, 14, 15, 19–21, 61, 230
elder peer counselor, 124
emergency preparedness, 37, 142–44
end–of–life preparation, 12, 83, 207–17, 230–34
entombment, 235
estate planning attorney, 10–16, 19, 20, 23, 26
ethical will. *See* legacy letter
ethics, 24, 225, 248
exercise, 135, 157, 158, 160–61, 163, 207

faith, 38, 82, 106, 125, 134, 225
falls. *See* hazards
family practitioner, 165, 166
Feldenkrais method practitioner, 170
fiduciary, 16, 19, 68, 70
finance/billing advocate, 199
financial advisor, 13, 43, 48, 58, 66, 67, 70–72
financial power of attorney. *See* durable power of attorney

fire prevention and safety, 143–44
Food Stamp Program. *See* Supplemental
  Nutrition Assistance Program
fraud, 43, 44, 49, 50–51, 54, 56, 144
funeral, 26, 55, 216–17, 235–44

Gawande, Atul, 164, 208, 231
Genworth Cost of Care. *See* cost of care
geriatric care manager. *See* aging life
  care manager
geriatric psychiatry hospitals, 202
geriatrician, 165
gerontologist, 272
geropsychologist, 272
gift giving, 46–48, 227
Gottlieb, Bill, 263
Green Houses. *See* Eden Alternative
guardianship, 12, 16, 18
guided autobiographer. *See* personal
  historian
gum inflammation, 186

hazards, reducing, 78, 100–102
HCPOA. *See* healthcare power of
  attorney
healthcare power of attorney, 14, 15, 16,
  17, 18, 23, 155, 176, 230, 247
Hindu, 227, 244, 245
HIPAA, 16, 19, 155, 172
hiring a homecare worker, 90–91, 93–97
home maintenance, 98–101, 194
home safe, 19
homeowner's insurance, 52, 59, 62–63,
  65
horticultural therapist, 170
hospice, 59, 84, 89, 91, 104, 106, 157,
  167, 181, 192, 193, 209–14, 216,
  217, 230, 231–32, 233, 250, 251
hospital stay, what to pack for, 175–76
hospitalist, 165, 167

identity theft. *See* scams
in–home helpers, 89–97
incapacity, 13, 15, 16, 22, 27
inheritance, 22, 24, 43

inpatient rehabilitation facilities, 104,
  195, 196–97
insurance, 26, 36, 39, 45, 52, 53, 55,
  58–66
internist, 165, 166
intestacy, 16, 17, 24
investment advisor, 44, 46, 48, 66, 67,
  69–78
investments, 36, 38–39, 43, 45–46
IRA. *See* retirement account
IRF. *See* inpatient rehabilitation
  facilities

Jewish, 244, 245
joint accounts, 45
junk, getting rid of, 137–42, 227

Kaddish, 245
kairos time, 232–33
keys, giving up. *See* transportation
  issues

labyrinths, 257–61
legacy letters, 226–27
Lewy Body dementia, 203
LGBT, 40, 41, 106, 110, 115, 145–46,
  242–43
liability insurance, 59, 65
life insurance, 63–64
living will. *See* advance directive
living with children, 82–85
location monitoring, 203
long–term care, 58, 59, 61, 65, 66, 105,
  181
LTC. *See* long–term care

Mabry, Rev. John, 252–53
Manteau–Rao, Marguerite, 206–7
MEDCottages, 87
Medicaid, 12, 19, 23–24, 61–62, 72,
  106, 109, 114, 115, 128, 154, 169,
  181, 182, 195, 211, 214; Medicaid
  beds 105
medical appointments, being prepared
  for, 173–75

medical emergency, 25
medical implants, 191–92
medical insurance, 59, 165, 168, 169, 180–83, 195, 211–14
medical specialists, 167–71
medically embedded devices, 24
Medicare, 39, 41, 49, 58, 59–62, 72, 89, 106, 128, 154, 161, 169, 180–82, 192, 195–97, 211–14
medications, 176–78; reminders/high–tech support, 176–77; disposing of medications, 177–78
Medigap insurance, 60, 171
meditation, 122, 157, 210, 234, 251, 257–61
memorial service, 217, 236–42
memory care facilities, 104–6, 108, 111–114, 116
memory gardens, 126–27
Miller, Kym Croft, 265
minimum required distribution, 42, 43
MRD. *See* minimum required distribution
music therapy, 127
Muslim, 244

naturally occurring retirement communities, 87
naturopathic doctor, 65
ND. *See* naturopathic doctor
need–based public benefit program. *See* Medicaid
NORC. *See* naturally occurring retirement communities
NP. *See* nurse practitioner
nurse practitioner, 165, 166, 171, 201
nursing homes, 58, 60, 61, 64, 65, 87, 104, 105, 109, 162, 170, 184, 185, 189, 193, 195, 196, 200, 211

obituary, 217, 241–42
occupational therapist, 130, 170, 171
ombudsman, 17, 85, 113, 114, 147
oncology considerations, related to dentistry, 187

oral fungal infections, 186
organ donation, 246–47

PA. *See* physician's assistant
pacemaker, 24, 192
palliative care, 213–14, 230, 251
Parkinson's disease, 203, 205–6
PCP. *See* primary care provider
pension, 39, 42, 64, 182
periodontal disease, 185–86
personal emergency response systems, 101–2
personal historian, 123, 127
personal representative, 15, 16, 17, 21, 25, 26
pets, 24, 90, 107, 110, 115, 136–37, 177, 204, 241
phishing scam. *See* scams
physcial therapist, 170
Physician Orders for Life–Sustaining Treatment. *See* POLST
physician's assistant, 89, 165, 166, 171
POA. *See* power of attorney
POD (paid on death) account, 45
POLST, 17, 18, 19, 24, 25, 154, 176, 208, 209, 230
post–death, 26–27, 215–17
power of attorney, 15–18, 25–26, 37, 155
prayers for the dead, 244–46
prescription drug coverage, 60–61, 181–82
Presence Care Project, 207
primary care provider, 165–67
probate, 13, 18, 22, 25, 26, 45
prosthodontist, 187
prothrombin time/prothrombin ratio/international normalized ratio, 190
psychiatric facilities, 202
PT/INR. *See* prothrombin time/prothrombin ratio/international normalized ratio
pulling–the–plug decision, 247–48

recurring payments, 52–53
renter's insurance, 59, 62–63

respite care, 212, 277
retirement accounts, 15, 41–43, 46
retirement income, 38, 39, 70
reverse mortgages, 57–58, 90, 100
Roman, Regina, 264
Roth IRA. *See r*etirement accounts

Sacred Dying Foundation, 234
safe deposit box, 19, 25, 27, 37, 238
safety. *See* emergency preparedness
salary, 39
same sex couple. *See* LGBT
same–sex relationship. *See* LGBT
scams, 48–51, 64, 79, 144–45
Scott, Paula Spencer, 137
self–care for caregivers, 206–7, 255–56
self–drafting legal documents, 13
Senior Health Insurance Benefits
    Assistance, 62, 72
senior move managers, 135, 137,
    141–42
shared housing, 79–81
SHIBA. *See* Senior Health Insurance
    Benefits Assistance
Sjögren's syndrome, 186
skilled nursing facilities, 104, 195, 196,
    197
sleep for elders, 101, 134, 157, 158,
    161, 168, 200, 206, 207, 214
SNAP. *See* Supplemental Nutrition
    Assistance Program
Social Security benefits, etc., 18, 27, 38,
    39–41, 49, 65, 72, 181
speech–language pathologist, 170–71
spiritual direction, 251–53
SSI. *See* Supplemental Security Income
stairlifts, 100

statutory document, 14
stockbrokers, 67, 70
storytelling, 127
strong box, 37
substance abuse, 159, 200
Supplemental Nutrition Assistance
    Program, 103
Supplemental Security Income, 181
symptom tracker, 173, 174

tax returns, 20, 26, 36, 40, 42, 48, 54,
    68
Thomas, Bill. *See* Eden Alternative
tiny houses, 87
transitions, 114, 130, 141, 197–201
transportation issues, 129–34
treasures, coping with, 136, 137–42,
    227–28
trusts, 12–18, 20, 21–25

umbrella insurance. *See* liability
    insurance
universal design, 102, 114, 115

vaccines, 178–79
vascular dementia, 203
Veriditas, 257–60
veterans, 59, 64, 72, 181, 182–83
vigiling, 232–34, 236, 239
Village to Village (VtV) Network, 86,
    87
village, 85–87, 124
virtual retirement community, 85–87
VRC. *See* virtual retirement community

wills, 14, 17, 21–22, 36
wisdom will. *See* legacy letter

Meet the Authors

Mary Jo Saavedra, MAIS, CMC, CAPS, CSA   Mary Jo is a practicing gerontologist and aging life care manager in Portland, Oregon. With a passion for empowering individuals of all ages to live their best lives, Mary Jo is dedicated to the holistic wellbeing of her clients. Using her six Pillars of Aging Wellbeing process, she helps elders choose how they will live with the challenges of aging; at the heart of every care or life plan she designs is respect for the needs and wants of the elder.

Mary Jo has additional certifications in aging-in-place, senior advising, and spiritual direction. An out-of-the-box thinker, she is credited with defining the conceptual model for an innovative real estate-focused rating system for classifying age-friendly homes. She is also an adjunct professor of gerontology at Marylhurst University, Pacific University, and Portland Community College; and she teaches aging and spirituality at the Franciscan Spiritual Center in Milwaukie, Oregon. In addition, Mary Jo has thirty years of professional experience across multiple industries including high tech, nonprofit, and health and wellbeing. More information can be found here: http://www.eldercare101book.com/.

Susan Cain McCarty, MAIS, CSA   Susan has a master's degree in interdisciplinary studies with a focus on gerontology and an undergraduate degree in communications. She also is a registered certified senior advisor and a member of the Society of Certified Senior Advisors, the American Society on Aging, and the Aging Life Care Association. Currently, Susan serves as an aging life care manager, advising older adults and/or their families about issues involving options for where to live, how to live safely, bringing help into one's home, creating new community, transportation, and many other topics. She also refers clients to healthcare, financial, and spiritual advisors who can help them as they age. In addition, Susan has been a professional marketer for over thirty years and has owned her own marketing consulting firm for over twenty years, providing services to high-tech companies. She also has been president of and managed a training company, providing training and consulting services to telcos.

Theresa Giddings, CPA, CFPR   Theresa is a senior move manager and a member of the National Association of Senior Move Managers (http://www.nasmm.org). As a senior move manager, she has extensive, practical knowledge about the costs, quality, and availability of various local community resources for elders. Theresa also is the founder of Soft Landings: Solutions for Seniors (http://www.softlandingsforseniors.com), an organization that offers specialized, compassionate move services for seniors and their families. Soft Landings also assists individuals who choose to stay in their homes. Well respected in her field, Theresa is a frequent speaker to senior groups, living communities, and real estate firms on "The Joy of Downsizing" and "Being Scamwise."

Theresa's senior move management business grew out of her over twenty-five years of being on the Portland Estate Planning Council and working in the fields of accounting and financial planning as a certified public accountant and a certified financial planner. She notes that, "With that background comes a profound commitment to connect with older adults and a desire to perform meaningful, trustworthy work. So, after helping many people achieve their retirement goals, I decided to assist them with their next transition in life."

Rev. Lawrence Hansen, MA, BCC/CFHPC, CT   Father Larry has worked in health care since 1987. He holds a bachelor's in English education from Oregon State University and a master's in Theology from the University of Portland. In 2000, Fr. Larry was ordained to the priesthood in the Catholic Apostolic Church in North America. He is board certified as a chaplain and fellow in hospice and palliative care with the College of Pastoral Supervision and Psychotherapy and holds the Certificate in Thanatology (CT) from the Association for Death Education and Counseling.

Currently, Fr. Larry serves as the associate chaplain at Kaiser Permanente, Kaiser Westside Medical Center in Hillsboro, Oregon. In addition, he teaches classes in the gerontology program at Portland Community College. He has given many lectures and presentations to students, healthcare professionals, and community groups. As a care provider, he has presided at hundreds of funerals for individuals from across a wide range of spiritual and religious traditions. In his spare time, Fr. Larry enjoys family activities and reading in theology, social science, and the humanities.

Dr. Benjamin B. Hellickson, DDS   Dr. Ben received his bachelor's degree in microbiology from Oregon State University and his Doctorate of Dental Surgery from the University of Pacific Arthur A. Dugoni School of Dentistry in San Francisco, California. He enjoys treating patients of all ages but finds treating the elder population especially rewarding. Currently, he practices dentistry at Mattson Hellickson Dental (http://www.mattsonhellicksondental. com) in Beaverton, Oregon.

Outside the office, Dr. Ben enjoys spending time with his wife, two dogs, and family. He has an active lifestyle and enjoys running, hiking, biking, surfing, skiing, and golfing. He often participates in running races and triathlons throughout the Pacific Northwest and California. An avid sports fan, Dr. Ben could very well be seen at many local football, baseball, and basketball games as well as cheering on the Portland Timbers!

Joyce Sjoberg, MA, RN, BSN, CMC   Joyce has a master's degree in organizational development and applied behavioral sciences from Bastyr University in Seattle as well as a bachelor's degree in nursing from Oregon Health Sciences University. She has over thirty years of experience caring for older adults and people with disabilities and is the owner of Aging Advisors. (http://www.agingadvisorspdx.com), a care management group. To provide holistic care for her clients and their entire family, Joyce draws from her nursing experience in acute hospital care, home health, hospice, and assisted living. She also draws from her experience teaching and training caregivers and consulting for various organizations. Her care focuses on the needs and desires of her clients and their families, and she is passionate about advocating on their behalf to support and create the living environment they want.

Joyce was a founding member of the Portland Professional Aging Life Care Association (ALCA). She is a certified member and has served as a co-chair of the Western Regional ALCA Conference. Joyce lives with her family and many pets in Portland, Oregon, where she is very involved in her community. She enjoys cooking, hiking, scrapbooking, bird watching, and singing.

Sara K. Yen, JD, LLM   Attorney Sara Yen focuses her practice (http:// www.yenlaw.com) on estate planning, elder law and Medicaid planning, special needs planning, and probate and estate administration. Her clients range from elders and boomers who need to do their own planning, to members of the Sandwich Generation who are dealing with the dual issues of caring for aging parents while still supporting their children. She also helps families plan to facilitate a higher quality of life for their children and family members with special needs.

Licensed to practice law in Oregon and Washington, Sara is a member of the Oregon State Bar Estate Planning, Elder Law, and Taxation Sections; Academy of Special Needs Planners; National Academy of Elder Law Attorneys; WealthCounsel; ElderCounsel; and Women in Insurance and Financial Services Portland Metro Chapter. Well respected in her field, she is a frequent speaker for attorneys, CPAs, and tax and financial professionals on estate planning, estate administration, elder law, and special needs planning. In her spare time, Sara enjoys family time with her husband and daughter, golfing, music, and cheering on the Portland Winterhawks.